101 Great Lowfat Pasta Dishes

101 Great Lowfat Pasta Dishes

Fast, Zesty & Healthful!

Margaret Martinez

PRIMA PUBLISHING

© 1996 by Margaret Martinez

PRIMA PUBLISHING and its colophon are trademarks of Prima
Communications, Inc.

Library of Congress Cataloging-in-Publication Data

Martinez, Margaret.
    101 great lowfat pasta dishes : fresh, zesty & healthful! /
by Margaret Martinez.
        p.   cm.
    Includes index.
    ISBN 0-7615-0414-1
    1. Cookery (Pasta)   2. Low-fat diet — Recipes.   I. Title.
TX809.M17M367   1996
641.8'22 — dc20   96-221
                                                                CIP

95 96 97 98 99 HH 10 9 8 7 6 5 4 3 2 1

Printed in the United States of America

Nutritional Analysis
A per serving nutritional breakdown is provided for each recipe. If a
range is given for an ingredient amount, the breakdown is based on
the smaller number. If a range is given for servings, the breakdown is
based on the larger number. If a choice of ingredients is given in an
ingredient listing, the breakdown is calculated using the first choice.
Nutritional content may vary depending on the specific brands or
types of ingredients used. "Optional" ingredients or those for which
no specific amount is stated are not included in the breakdown.
Nutritional figures are rounded to the nearest whole number.

How to Order:
Single copies may be ordered from Prima Publishing, P.O. Box 1260,
Rocklin, CA 95677; telephone (916) 632-4400. Quantity discounts are
available. On your letterhead, include information concerning the in-
tended use of the books and the number of books you wish to purchase.

To my husband for his tremendous love, encouragement, and assistance thoughout the writing of this cookbook.

To my grandmothers, mother, father, brother, and all my relatives who always give me their love, support, and encouragement in the attainment of personal goals.

To my Aunt Tony, a gifted cook, who fostered my special pride in cooking.

To Alice Anderson, for her faithful support as my editor.

Contents

Quick and Delicious Light Pasta Sauces 45

Light Pasta Dishes with Pizazz 83

Now You're Cooking Main Pasta Dishes   143

Hot Baked Dishes in Minutes   195

Introduction

I am dedicating these 101 great lowfat recipes to pasta lovers everywhere. This cookbook is for all of you who enjoy a plateful of warm, sweet-smelling, chewy pasta. It is up to you to choose how you like your pasta served best: smothered in a special creamy sauce, "al dente" with fresh herbs and vegetables, or saturated with succulent pieces of meat. However you choose, I know you will enjoy preparing and using these original and flavorful lowfat pasta dishes.

Used around the world, pasta is a popular ingredient found in many healthful international cuisines. Few other foods have the versatility or universal appeal of the simple noodle. Made from a variety of shapes, sizes, and ingredients, pasta tastes delicious, is nutritious, and enhances any meal. Pasta is also economical and widely eaten by health enthusiasts for carbohydrates that provide an excellent source of energy. A new generation of pasta lovers is finding inspiration from the multiflavored pasta now available in most large supermarkets. Throughout the United States you will find different types of pasta made with eggs, flour, herbs, vegetables, and other superb flavors. More than 100 varieties of pasta are now available in the United States and over 600 varieties exist worldwide. The various shapes and textures are important and absorb different flavors from the ingredients into the pasta. Thin or small pastas are best for soups and salads, while the larger, thicker pastas and shells are best with rich tomato or creamy sauces.

If you love pasta, you'll find this book rewarding to use. It is packed with appealing recipes using fresh ingredients and offering different kinds of low-calorie ideas for easy-to-prepare pasta dishes. It might even surprise you to discover so many recipes for appetizing dishes that are also low in fat and calories. The secret is always in the ingredients and how you prepare them. Thankfully, food manufacturers are quickly responding to consumer demand and new dietary trends. Every day new varieties of low- and nonfat products are appearing on the market. These products provide health-conscious cooks with the special items necessary to make their nutritious dishes without losing texture or appeal. You can count on the flavor in these pasta recipes — and even not mind losing the extra calories, fat, and cholesterol.

Super Good Pasta Starters

The first section, *Super Good Pasta Starters*, offers an enticing collection of delicious and attractive salads and soups. Fresh vegetables, fruits, herbs, and other seasonings blend to give a distinctive flavor to each dish. Red, ripe tomatoes, green and yellow onions, yellow pineapples, black beans, and small bunches of aromatic herbs are pleasing additions to salads and soups made with pasta.

The salad recipes present low-calorie, versatile salads that are great as a light main course for lunch, a side dish, or even a late-night snack. These luscious, attractive salads subtly reveal the presence of many special ingredients. Made in minutes, the salads stimulate the senses, warm and soothe the appetite, or set the stage for the delicious meal to follow.

Good soup is often an important part of a satisfying, fulfilling meal. Soups in this section are homespun, nutritious concoctions that display a colorful array of piquant, enticing flavors and chewy textures. A hot, steaming bowl of hearty, fragrant soup is heavenly on a cold, snowy afternoon or appetizing as a stimulating starter for an elegant meal. In a cup or small bowl, you can also appreciate these thick, savory soups as a late-night snack.

Quick and Delicious Light Pasta Sauces

Sauces are fundamental to the pasta diet and often reveal the true essence of classical cuisine. If you like to cook with pasta, you should always have your favorite sauce in your collection of recipes. Served warm, thick or thin, red or white, sauces enliven your pasta meals with unforgettable elegance, color, flair, and appetizing flavor. Choose a delicious sauce and transform a plateful of pasta into an exceptional masterpiece with contrasting flavors, aromas, textures, and colors.

The *Quick and Delicious Light Pasta Sauces* section contains a variety of new and traditional sauces to use with your choice of pasta. These sauce recipes offer enthusiastic cooks an array of satisfying choices: the spicy, rich taste of tomato sauce, the subtle flavor of a delicate herb sauce, or the rich smoothness of a creamy sauce. With these low-calorie and lowfat recipes, you too can concoct magical potions to impress your family and friends. Refreshing, tingly, rich, spicy, mouth-watering, and satisfying, these versatile sauces proudly proclaim their own unique exquisiteness.

Light Pasta Dishes with Pizazz

The recipes in the *Light Pasta Dishes with Pizazz* section offer opportunities to enjoy light cooking with pasta and an assortment of fresh, colorful ingredients. Savor the enticing flavors and textures, confident in the knowledge that the pasta dishes are nutritious, low-calorie, and always satisfying.

Prepared with a medley of vegetables, seafood, herbs, and sauces, these pasta dishes demonstrate the quintessential versatility of the much-honored noodle. The recipes present tempting international cuisine, including a palette of traditional Italian, spicy Southwestern, exotic Mediterranean, and mystical Oriental dishes. Try these international accents to create your next great lunch or dinner. Make them in advance, microwave them when you are ready to eat, and enjoy the light, delicious meals at your leisure.

Now You're Cooking Main Pasta Dishes

The pasta dishes in the *Now You're Cooking Main Pasta Dishes* section are bursting with robust flavor and appeal. Beef and poultry lovers will discover a variety of appetizing ideas and enjoy cooking these lowfat, low-calorie recipes. Using a variety of sauces, vegetables, and other savory ingredients with beef or poultry, you can easily change a simple dish into an enticing course of heavenly fare.

Everyone appreciates a hearty, homespun meal especially when served with a plateful of warm, luscious pasta. Whether you grill, stew, bake, broil, stir-fry, or microwave, these main dishes are fast, delicious, and always nutritious. You do not have to look far for a favorite recipe that you can feature as a tempting main course for your family and friends. Use these pasta recipes to create a visual feast of flavor and nutrition.

Hot Baked Pasta Dishes in Minutes

If you are looking to cut your cooking time in half, begin by looking in the *Hot Baked Pasta Dishes in Minutes* section. Busy cooks who need to get their meals to the table in minutes will appreciate these recipes. When there are not enough hours in the day, prepare these dishes in advance, refrigerate them, and after a busy day, offer healthful meals in just a few minutes.

The different cuisines around the world present many thousands of ways to prepare casseroles using different varieties of pastas. The recipes in this section are an array of simple pasta dishes baked with vegetables, fruits, poultry, beef, seafood, and other appealing ingredients. Such specialities are especially appealing when skillfully combined with a fresh array of herbs, savory sauces, and other seasonings.

Pasta is the perfect choice any way you choose to prepare it. Enjoy reading and experimenting with the recipes found in this cookbook. It is a tempting selection of ideas showing you, the busy cook, how to turn a simple pasta dish into an extraordinary, happy event. Cook and discover new ways to adapt these pasta dishes to suit your own unique taste and cooking style. Now you too can prepare 101 great lowfat pasta dishes in the comfort of your own kitchen. I hope you enjoy presenting your new, irresistible creations to your family, friends, and other special guests. Happy Cooking!

Cooking Hints and Recipe Notes

In this section I have included information about the recipes and a few cooking tips to help you create the perfect pasta meal. These are recipes that will have your family and friends singing your praises.

Cooking with Pasta and Other Ingredients

- Cook the pasta until it is al dente. This means that the pasta is tender but still firm or chewy to the teeth. Do not overcook pasta or it will become mushy and very unpleasant tasting.
- Drain cooked pasta in a colander.
- You can refrigerate cooked pasta in a tightly sealed container for three to five days.
- If you want to freeze the pasta dish, prepare the pasta in a baked recipe, such as lasagne or a tuna casserole, before freezing.
- To bake a frozen pasta dish, thaw the dish to room temperature before baking as directed in the recipe.
- Keep pasta and sauces separate while storing overnight or longer in the refrigerator.
- Fresh eggplant can have a somewhat bitter taste when eaten. To reduce the bitterness, slice the eggplant and lay the slices on paper towels. Lightly salt the eggplant slices to draw the juices to the surface. After 10 to 20 minutes, wipe the excess moisture off the surface with a paper towel.
- Nothing can replace the distinct, pungent flavor of fresh herbs. Nowadays, to save time and for convenience, our

7

inclination is to use the dried herbs sold in containers on grocery shelves. If you do not already use fresh herbs, I urge you to try using them whenever possible. Fresh herbs contribute a wonderful, earthy flavor and rich color to every dish. Try a taste test to discover if you can tell the difference in the flavors between fresh and dried herbs.

- Broth appears in the list of recipe ingredients in this cookbook. For best results, use homemade broth made with herbs, vegetables, chicken, or beef. Chill, then skim the broth to remove any fat. As an alternative, you can use the low-sodium, fat-free chicken, vegetable, or beef broth that you can buy in jars or cans.

- Apple cider vinegar often appears as a recipe ingredient. Feel free to experiment with different types of vinegars to add new flavors to your pasta dishes. Flavored vinegars, such as tarragon, balsamic, and red wine vinegar, are just a few kinds of an enticing array of choices.

About the Recipes:

- The recipes in this cookbook offer a range of spiciness that is generally very mild to spicy in flavor. For example, measurements, such as 1 to 3 cloves garlic, 2 to 4 sprigs fresh parsley, or 1/2 to 1 anaheim chile, will show possible amounts that you can use in food preparation. The level of spiciness for each dish is left up to you, the cook in charge. If you like milder foods, use the low end of the range or less. If you like spicy foods, use the high end of the range or more. Once you try the recipes, I urge you to adapt the quantity of fresh herbs and chiles according to your personal tastes.

- If the recipe calls for tomato sauce, you can select from the several recipes presented in the *Quick and Delicious Light Pasta Sauces* section. This section offers an assortment of tomato-based sauces, including Spicy Mexican-Style

Tomato Sauce (recipe # 18), Italian-Style Tomato Sauce (recipe # 19), Chunky Marinara Sauce (recipe # 24), and Primavera Sauce (recipe # 28).

About the Nutritional Information:

- Each recipe includes a table showing the estimated nutritional information for the combination of ingredients used in each recipe. In these tables, food values have been rounded up and trace amounts listed as zero. Actual figures may vary slightly depending on the brands of the products and actual amounts of ingredients used to prepare the recipes.

- All the recipes in this cookbook feature limited amounts of fat and less than 300 calories per serving.

Super Good
Pasta Starters

1

—❦—

Chicken Paprika Salad

Preparation time: 15 minutes

Pineapples sweetly embellish the tart, refreshing flavor of
this colorful, festive chicken salad. If you prefer, you can
substitute turkey, beef, or grilled chicken to create another
tasty, hearty version. Serve this salad as the perfect light
luncheon or use more modest portions for smaller dinner
salads.

1/4 cup (about 1/2 ounce) dry fideo pasta, cooked according
    to package directions, drained, and rinsed
1/2 cup finely sliced green onions
3/4 cup cooked chicken chunks (about 6 ounces)
1/2 cup pineapple chunks
1/3 cup pineapple juice
1 tablespoon lime juice
1 cup small mushroom caps, sliced in half
1/2 small red bell pepper, finely sliced into 2-inch pieces
1/2 small yellow bell pepper, finely sliced into 2-inch pieces
1 to 2 teaspoons minced fresh marjoram leaves
Salt and freshly ground pepper
1/2 bunch (6 ounces) spinach, cleaned and torn into pieces
    (about 2 cups)
1 small tomato, halved and cut into 8 to 12 slices
Dash of paprika

Combine all the ingredients, excluding the salt, pepper, spinach, tomato, and paprika in a large bowl. Salt and pepper the salad according to individual taste. Toss in the spinach leaves. Drain the salad mixture; reserve the marinade. Arrange equal portions of the salad mixture on six salad plates. Garnish each salad plate with the tomato slices and paprika. Sprinkle the remaining marinade over each salad.

6 servings

Each serving provides:

85	Calories	20 g	Carbohydrate
13 g	Protein	59 mg	Sodium
1 g	Fat	24 mg	Cholesterol

2

New Mexico Pasta Salad

Preparation time: 15 minutes

Cilantro, corn, and black beans are colorful Southwestern favorites. Mixed with pasta, this interesting combination adds pleasing flavor and texture to the salad. For an interesting variation, try garbanzo or red beans in place of the black beans. If you need to prepare the salad in advance for picnics or buffets, store the salad in a tightly sealed container and refrigerate overnight.

1½ cups (about 3 ounces) dry salad pasta, cooked according to package directions, drained, and rinsed
½ cup finely sliced green onions
½ small red onion, diced
1 cup corn, cooked
½ cup cooked black beans
2 small tomatoes, chopped
½ small red bell pepper, diced
½ small fresh anaheim chile, seeded, washed, and finely diced (optional, for a spicier dish)
3 tablespoons lowfat mayonnaise
Salt and freshly ground pepper
¼ cup chopped black olives
1 to 2 sprigs fresh cilantro, minced (optional)
¼ to 1 teaspoon chopped red chile pepper flakes (optional, for a spicier dish)

Combine all the ingredients, excluding the salt, pepper, olives, cilantro, and chile pepper flakes in a medium-size bowl. Salt and pepper the salad according to individual taste. Serve equal portions of the salad on five salad plates. Garnish with the olives, cilantro, and chile pepper flakes.

5 servings

	Each serving provides:		
149	Calories	31 g	Carbohydrate
5 g	Protein	115 mg	Sodium
1 g	Fat	0 mg	Cholesterol

3

---🦋---

Supreme Layered-Pasta Salad

Preparation time: 20 minutes

Layered salads are an exceptionally enticing feast of
fresh, colorful ingredients. Serve this salad in a large glass
salad bowl for extra eye-appeal. The festive layers, visible
through the glass, will charmingly appeal to hungry diners
and naturally elicit the coveted oohs and ahhs of apprecia-
tion from your guests. For a colorful variation and extra
flavor, try adding pineapples, corn, or lime juice.

$\frac{1}{2}$ small head romaine lettuce (6 ounces), cleaned and torn
    into pieces (about 2 cups)
1 cup (about 2 ounces) dry salad shell pasta, cooked ac-
    cording to package directions, drained, and rinsed
1 small carrot, grated
1 cup fresh peas or snow peas, cooked
$\frac{1}{3}$ cup nonfat mayonnaise
8 broccoli florets
$\frac{1}{2}$ small red onion, finely diced
1 cup sliced mushrooms
$\frac{1}{2}$ small red bell pepper, halved and cut into julienne strips
$\frac{1}{2}$ cup nonfat cottage cheese

1 medium-size ripe tomato, chopped
2 tablespoons grated lowfat mozzarella or Swiss cheese
1/4 cup sliced black olives
1/2 cup finely sliced green onions
4 fresh basil leaves, minced
Salt and freshly ground pepper

In the order shown, layer each of the ingredients, excluding the basil leaves, salt, and pepper in a large, glass salad bowl. Extend the salad ingredients to the side of the bowl so that the colorful layers appear through the glass. Garnish the salad with the basil leaves. Salt and pepper according to individual taste.

8 servings

Each serving provides:

130	Calories	24 g	Carbohydrate
5 g	Protein	721 mg	Sodium
1 g	Fat	3 mg	Cholesterol

4

Curry Shrimp Salad

Preparation time: 20 minutes

This attractive seafood salad offers sophisticated flavors and aromas that will naturally appeal to shrimp lovers. Succulent shrimp combines with fresh, crunchy vegetables and the tantalizing flavor of curry. For extra flavor, add one to two teaspoons of extra-virgin olive oil (40 calories per teaspoon). Instead of using shrimp, try substituting crab, scallops, or octopus to create other attractive variations of this exotic garden fresh salad.

½ cup (about 1 ounce) dry salad pasta, cooked according
    to package directions, drained, and rinsed
½ pound fresh shrimp, peeled, deveined, and cleaned
½ cup fresh snow peas
1 tablespoon water
1 tablespoon lime juice
1 tablespoon apple cider vinegar
1 teaspoon curry powder
1 small tomato, chopped
½ cup finely sliced green onions
⅓ small red bell pepper, finely diced
1 to 2 sprigs fresh celery leaves, minced
1 to 2 teaspoons minced fresh tarragon leaves
½ small head romaine lettuce (6 ounces), cleaned and torn
    into pieces (about 2 cups)
Salt and freshly ground pepper

In a saucepan, bring 2 cups of water to a boil; reduce the heat to low. Add the shrimp and snow peas to the boiling water; the water should barely cover the shrimp. Simmer the shrimp for 3 to 4 minutes until the shrimp turns pink. Drain the shrimp and snow peas; set aside.

Combine the water, lime juice, vinegar, and curry powder in a bowl. Stir in the shrimp, snow peas, pasta, tomato, onions, bell pepper, celery, and tarragon. Place the lettuce on six salad plates. Arrange a portion of the shrimp mixture on top of each plate. Salt and pepper the salads according to individual taste.

6 servings

Each serving provides:

118	Calories	8 g	Carbohydrate
19 g	Protein	45 mg	Sodium
1 g	Fat	35 mg	Cholesterol

5

Mediterranean Garden Salad

Preparation time: 20 minutes
Marinade time: 10 to 15 minutes

The garbanzo beans in this zesty salad provide lots of protein. The Parmesan cheese, tangy salad dressing, and fresh herbs offer their own special blend of flavors. Serve this light, refreshing salad as a starter before dinner or as a late-night snack. For other special toppings, try sprinkling the salad with feta or other chunky cheeses, black olives, or cooked black beans.

½ cup (about 1 ounce) dry rotini or salad pasta, cooked
    according to package directions, drained, and rinsed
1 teaspoon apple cider vinegar
1 teaspoon extra-virgin olive oil
1 tablespoon lemon juice
1 to 2 teaspoons minced fresh dill weed
1 teaspoon Dijon-style mustard
1 tablespoon grated nonfat Parmesan cheese
½ small red onion, halved and finely sliced
1 cup cooked garbanzo beans
½ small red bell pepper, diced
6 cherry tomatoes, washed, and halved
½ cup finely sliced green onions

¹/₂ small head romaine lettuce (6 ounces), cleaned and torn
    into pieces (about 2 cups)
1 medium-size egg, hard-cooked and diced
Salt and freshly ground pepper

Combine the vinegar, oil, lemon juice, dill, mustard,
Parmesan cheese, and red onion in a medium-size bowl.
Add the pasta, beans, bell pepper, tomatoes, and onions.
Marinate the salad ingredients in the refrigerator for 10 to
15 minutes. Arrange the lettuce on six salad plates. Serve the
pasta mixture on each plate of lettuce. Garnish each salad
with the egg. Salt and pepper according to individual taste.

6 servings

Each serving provides:

89	Calories	14 g	Carbohydrate
5 g	Protein	73 mg	Sodium
2 g	Fat	32 mg	Cholesterol

6

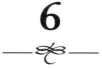

Tropical Fruit Salad

Preparation time: 15 minutes
Refrigeration time: 10 minutes

Fruit lovers will enjoy the sweet, delicate flavors found in this festive, yet simple fruit salad. A fruit salad is especially pleasing before a spicy or hearty pasta meal. If you need to prepare your meal ahead of time, this large salad refrigerates and stores well for a few hours in a tightly sealed container.

1 ounce dry angel hair pasta, cooked according to package
    directions, drained, and rinsed
1/4 cup lime juice
1/2 cup pineapple juice
1/2 cup sliced banana (about 1 medium)
1 cup sliced mango (1-inch pieces)
1 cup sliced pineapple (1-inch pieces)
1 cup sliced papaya (1-inch pieces)
1 orange or tangerine, peeled and sectioned
1/2 bunch (6 ounces) spinach, cleaned and torn into pieces
    (about 2 cups)

Combine all the ingredients, excluding the spinach, in a medium-size bowl. Cover; refrigerate the salad for 10 minutes. Drain the fruit and reserve the marinade. Place the spinach leaves on six salad plates. Decoratively arrange the fruit salad on each salad plate. Drizzle the reserved marinade over the individual salads.

6 servings

Each serving provides:

103	Calories	28 g	Carbohydrate
2 g	Protein	18 mg	Sodium
1 g	Fat	0 mg	Cholesterol

7

—❧—

Tuna and Celery Pasta Salad

Preparation time: 15 minutes

Tuna and celery are the featured ingredients in this colorful, attractive salad nested on a bed of fresh romaine lettuce leaves. If you prefer, you can use any firm white fish
or seafood in place of the tuna in this recipe. For other interesting variations, try adding a hard-cooked egg or ten-
derly cooked florets of broccoli or cauliflower as a special,
colorful topping.

1 1/2 cups (about 3 ounces) dry macaroni pasta, cooked ac-
    cording to package directions, drained, and rinsed
1 cup (about 1/2 pound) cooked fresh tuna chunks (1-inch
    pieces)
1 teaspoon lemon juice
1/2 cup nonfat mayonnaise
1/2 small red bell pepper, finely diced
1/2 cup finely sliced celery
1 to 2 sprigs fresh celery leaves, minced
Salt and freshly ground pepper
1/2 small head romaine lettuce (6 ounces), cleaned and torn
    into pieces (about 2 cups)
6 cherry tomatoes
1/2 cup finely sliced green onions
1/4 cup diced black olives

Combine the pasta, tuna, lemon juice, mayonnaise, bell pepper, celery, and celery leaves in a medium-size bowl. Salt
and pepper the dish according to individual taste.

Place the lettuce on six salad plates. Arrange the
tuna salad mixture on each plate. Attractively arrange the
cherry tomatoes on top of each salad. Garnish the salads
with the green onions and olives.

6 servings

Each serving provides:

122	Calories	16 g	Carbohydrate
11 g	Protein	217 mg	Sodium
1 g	Fat	18 mg	Cholesterol

8

---&---

Pineapple and Pork Pasta Salad

Preparation time: 15 minutes

This is a favorite easy, make-ahead salad packed with flavor and nutrition. It includes ingredients from each of the essential food groups. You will enjoy serving this impressive salad at picnics, buffets, or potluck occasions. Served with toasted multigrain bread, this exotic, tempting salad is perfect for a light luncheon. For extra appeal and nutrition, serve this delicious salad over a bed of fresh spinach.

½ cup (about 1 ounce) dry salad or shell pasta, cooked according to package directions, drained, and rinsed
½ cup cooked pork loin pieces (1-inch strips)
½ cup sliced green onions
½ small red bell pepper, finely diced
1 cup crushed pineapple
¼ cup pineapple juice
1 small carrot, grated
1 to 2 sprigs fresh celery leaves, minced
⅓ cup nonfat mayonnaise
Salt and freshly ground pepper
Dash of paprika

Combine all the ingredients, excluding the salt, pepper, and paprika in a medium-size bowl. Salt and pepper the dish according to individual taste. Arrange the salad on four salad plates. Garnish each salad with a dash of paprika.

4 servings

Each serving provides:

131	Calories	26 g	Carbohydrate
10 g	Protein	218 mg	Sodium
2 g	Fat	22 mg	Cholesterol

9

—❧—

Classic Macaroni Salad

Preparation time: 15 minutes

Do not give up your favorite pasta salads with mayonnaise just because they have too many calories or too much fat. Macaroni salad lovers will enjoy this salad recipe as a satisfying salad with tangy flavors and eye-catching colors. Make this classic salad the night before to give the flavors time to blend. For a colorful variation, add a diced, hard-cooked egg, pineapple chunks, paprika, parsley, or red onions as an attractive topping.

2 cups (about 4 ounces) dry small macaroni pasta, cooked
     according to package directions, drained, and rinsed
1/2 cup finely sliced green onions
1 small celery stalk, finely diced
1 small carrot, grated
1/2 cup nonfat mayonnaise
1 tablespoon pineapple juice
2 teaspoons Dijon-style mustard
1 to 2 sprigs fresh celery leaves, minced
1 to 2 teaspoons minced fresh sage
Salt and freshly ground pepper

Combine all the ingredients except the salt and pepper in a medium-size bowl. Salt and pepper the dish according to individual taste. Arrange the salad on six salad plates.

6 servings

Each serving provides:			
96	Calories	20 g	Carbohydrate
3 g	Protein	224 mg	Sodium
0 g	Fat	0 mg	Cholesterol

10

_꧁—_

Tomato Alphabet Soup

Preparation time: 15 minutes
Cooking time: 10 minutes

This special soup gets its hearty, zesty flavor from a spicy
concoction of tomatoes. Simmered with the flavor of
tomatoes, chiles, and herbs, this satisfying soup has eye
and taste bud appeal. For even more color and flavor, add
corn kernels, yellow bell peppers, or cilantro to the soup.

$\frac{1}{2}$ small yellow onion, thickly sliced
$\frac{1}{2}$ cup finely sliced green onions
1 to 2 cloves garlic, crushed in a garlic press
$\frac{1}{2}$ small green bell pepper, diced
1 medium-size ripe tomato, blanched, peeled, and diced
3 cups tomato sauce
4 cups low-sodium beef broth
$\frac{1}{4}$ cup uncooked alphabet pasta
1 to 2 teaspoons minced fresh oregano leaves
1 to 2 teaspoons minced fresh sage
Salt and freshly ground pepper
1 to 3 sprigs minced fresh parsley (optional)

Heat a 5-quart pot over medium-high heat. Sauté the yellow and green onions, garlic, bell pepper, and tomato until the onions are tender.

Stir in the tomato sauce, broth, pasta, oregano, and sage. Bring the soup to a boil; reduce the heat to low. Simmer the soup for 10 minutes. Salt and pepper according to individual taste. Serve the hot soup garnished with the parsley.

4 servings

Each serving provides:

82	Calories	18 g	Carbohydrate
3 g	Protein	30 mg	Sodium
1 g	Fat	0 mg	Cholesterol

11

_❧_

Chicken and Fideo Soup

Preparation time: 15 minutes
Cooking time: 7 to 10 minutes

Use leftover chicken in this recipe to transform a popular,
home-cooked soup into a zippy, hearty combination of
chicken and fideo noodles. Freshly made, this delicious
soup easily multiplies into larger portions or adds delightful flair to a small lunch or dinner. Serve the soup with
lemon or lime wedges for an added exotic twist of flavor.

1 small yellow onion, quartered and finely sliced
^{1}/$_2$ cup finely sliced green onions
1 to 2 cloves garlic, diced
^{1}/$_2$ cup sliced celery
6 cherry tomatoes, sliced
1 cup (^{1}/$_2$ pound) shredded, cooked, extra-lean chicken
^{1}/$_2$ cup (about 1 ounce) uncooked fideo pasta
3 cups water
3 cups low-sodium chicken broth
1 to 2 teaspoons minced fresh oregano leaves
1 to 2 sprigs fresh thyme
Salt and freshly ground pepper
1 to 3 sprigs fresh parsley or cilantro, minced (optional)

Heat a 5-quart pot over medium-high heat. Sauté the yellow and green onions, garlic, celery, and tomatoes until the onions are tender; stir frequently.

Stir in the chicken, pasta, water, broth, oregano, and thyme. Bring the soup to a boil; reduce the heat to low. Cover; simmer until the pasta is just tender (al dente), about 7 to 10 minutes. Salt and pepper the soup according to individual taste. Remove the thyme before serving. Serve the hot soup garnished with the parsley or cilantro.

6 servings

Each serving provides:

91	Calories	8 g	Carbohydrate
12 g	Protein	45 mg	Sodium
1 g	Fat	32 mg	Cholesterol

12

— ✣ —

Clam Bisque

Preparation time: 10 minutes
Cooking time: 10 to 15 minutes

This savory and nourishing clam soup is a fabulous blend
of rich flavors that excite the taste buds. The tantalizing
flavors of the clams, garlic, and onions simmer together to
create a healthful, mouth-watering soup. Add a dash of
nutmeg or diced green chiles for a subtle flavor variation.

1 small yellow onion, chopped
$1/2$ cup sliced green onions
1 to 2 cloves garlic, minced
$1/2$ pound fresh clam meat
$1/4$ cup uncooked small shell pasta
4 teaspoons flour
$1^1/2$ cups nonfat milk
1 cup water
1 cup low-sodium chicken broth
1 cup nonfat sour cream
$1/4$ cup clam juice
1 to 2 sprigs fresh thyme
Salt and freshly ground pepper
1 to 3 sprigs fresh parsley, minced (optional)

Heat a large saucepan over medium-high heat. Sauté the yellow and green onions, garlic, and clam meat until the onions are tender; stir frequently. Combine the pasta, flour, milk, water, broth, sour cream, clam juice, and thyme in a medium-size bowl; mix well.

Stir the milk mixture into the saucepan; stir constantly until the sauce thickens. Reduce the heat to low. Simmer for 10 to 15 minutes. Salt and pepper the dish according to individual taste. Remove the thyme before serving. Serve the hot soup garnished with the parsley.

4 servings

		Each serving provides:		
154	Calories	33 g	Carbohydrate
16 g	Protein	189 mg	Sodium
1 g	Fat	22 mg	Cholesterol

13

⸘

Spicy Minestrone Soup

Preparation time: 15 minutes
Cooking time: 12 to 15 minutes

This easy-to-prepare adaption of a traditional Italian soup, offers an unbeatable combination of tomatoes, herbs, and vegetables. For extra flavor, garnish the soup with nonfat Parmesan cheese. Served with a chunk of bread and a fresh garden salad, this soup provides a particularly appetizing and satisfying luncheon.

1 small yellow onion, chopped
1/2 cup finely sliced green onions
1 to 2 cloves garlic, crushed in a garlic press
1/2 small green bell pepper, diced
1 small carrot, finely sliced
4 medium-size ripe tomatoes, blanched or roasted, peeled, seeded, and finely chopped
1/4 cup cooked red or garbanzo beans
4 1/2 cups low-sodium beef broth
1 to 2 sprigs fresh thyme
1 to 2 teaspoons minced fresh oregano leaves
1 bay leaf
1/2 cup uncooked small shell pasta
Salt and freshly ground pepper
1 to 3 sprigs fresh parsley, minced (optional)

Heat a 5-quart pot over medium-high heat. Sauté the yellow and green onions, garlic, bell pepper, carrot, and tomatoes until the onions are tender. Stir in the beans, broth, thyme, oregano, and bay leaf. Bring the soup to a boil; reduce the heat to low. Add the pasta shells.

Simmer the soup until the noodles soften (al dente), about 12 to 15 minutes. Salt and pepper the soup according to individual taste. Remove the bay leaf and thyme before serving. Serve the hot soup garnished with the parsley.

6 servings

Each serving provides:

71	Calories	15 g	Carbohydrate
3 g	Protein	19 mg	Sodium
1 g	Fat	0 mg	Cholesterol

14

Seafood and Rotini Bisque

Preparation time: 15 minutes
Cooking time: 15 to 20 minutes

Why not start your next meal with this savory seafood soup? For an unusual first course appetizer, this delicious combination of fresh seafood stimulates and prepares the taste buds for the meal to come. For the perfect hearty lunch, serve this soup piping hot with a chunk of French bread and a small macaroni salad.

1 small yellow onion, quartered and finely sliced
½ cup finely sliced green onions
1 to 3 cloves garlic, minced
1 small celery stalk with leaves, diagonally sliced
4 small ripe tomatoes, blanched or roasted, peeled, seeded, and coarsely chopped
1 cup (½ pound) assorted fresh seafood pieces, cleaned (firm white fish, scallops, shrimp, or clams), (about 1½-inch chunks)
2 teaspoons lime juice
1 cup low-sodium chicken broth
3 cups water
½ cup uncooked rotini or rotelle pasta

1 to 2 sprigs fresh thyme
1 to 2 teaspoons minced fresh basil leaves
1 bay leaf
1 to 2 teaspoons minced fresh oregano leaves
Salt and freshly ground pepper
4 sprigs fresh parsley or cilantro (optional)

Heat a large 5-quart pot over medium-high heat. Sauté the yellow and green onions, garlic, celery, tomatoes, and seafood pieces until the celery is tender; stir frequently. Stir in the lime juice, broth, and water. Bring the soup to a boil; reduce the heat to low.

Stir in the pasta, thyme, basil, bay leaf, and oregano. Cover; simmer gently for 15 to 20 minutes. Salt and pepper the dish according to individual taste. Remove the thyme and bay leaf before serving. Serve the hot soup garnished with the parsley or cilantro sprigs.

4 servings

Each serving provides:

63	Calories	8 g	Carbohydrate
8 g	Protein	62 mg	Sodium
1 g	Fat	22 mg	Cholesterol

15

—❦—

Meatball Alphabet Soup

Preparation time: 10 minutes
Cooking time: 45 to 60 minutes

This savory, nourishing meatball soup is a fabulous blend of rich flavors and appealing colors. The tantalizing, simmered flavors of the meat and tomatoes present a filling, mouth-watering one-dish meal. This traditional specialty is quick and easy to prepare and especially delicious on a cold or rainy day. To reduce fat and cholesterol, try substituting the required fresh egg with a whole egg substitute.

³/₄ pound extra-lean ground round beef (about 1¹/₂ cups)
1 medium-size egg, lightly beaten
¹/₄ cup uncooked alphabet pasta
1 medium-size yellow onion, finely sliced
1 to 2 cloves garlic, minced
¹/₄ to 1 small fresh anaheim chile, seeded, washed, and
    finely diced (optional, for a spicier dish)
3 medium-size ripe tomatoes, blanched or roasted, peeled,
    and diced
2 cups low-sodium beef broth
5 cups water
1 to 2 teaspoons minced fresh oregano leaves
2 bay leaves
1 to 2 sprigs fresh thyme
Salt and freshly ground pepper

Combine the meat, egg, and pasta in a medium-size bowl. Roll the meat mixture into 1 ½-inch balls; set aside. Heat a 5-quart pot over medium-high heat. Sauté the onion, garlic, anaheim chile, and tomatoes until the onions are tender; stir frequently.

Stir in the broth, water, oregano, bay leaves, and thyme; combine well. Bring the soup to a boil and gently drop the meatballs in the pot. Reduce the heat to low. Cover; simmer the soup for 45 to 60 minutes. Skim off any excess fat. Salt and pepper the dish according to individual taste. Remove the bay leaves and thyme before serving. Serve the hot soup in individual bowls.

6 servings

	Each serving provides:		
171	Calories	14 g	Carbohydrate
20 g	Protein	61 mg	Sodium
4 g	Fat	71 mg	Cholesterol

16

—✧—

Broccoli and Angel Hair
Pasta Soup

Preparation time: 10 minutes
Cooking time: 15 to 20 minutes

This flavorful, garden-fresh soup presents the specially-
blended flavors of broccoli, carrots, and tomatoes to subtle
perfection. Nutritious and satisfyingly filling, this soup
recipe offers a unique, delicious combination for lovers of
hearty vegetable soups.

1 small yellow onion, finely sliced
½ cup finely sliced green onions
1 to 2 cloves garlic, crushed in a garlic press
8 broccoli florets, halved (about 1 cup)
1 small carrot, pared and thinly sliced
1 small ripe tomato, peeled and finely diced
¼ cup (about ½ ounce) broken, uncooked
　　angel hair pasta
2 cups low-sodium chicken broth
4 cups water
1 cup tomato sauce
1 to 2 teaspoons minced fresh oregano leaves
1 bay leaf
Salt and freshly ground pepper
2 to 4 sprigs fresh parsley or cilantro, minced (optional)

Heat a large saucepan over medium-high heat. Sauté the yellow and green onions, garlic, broccoli, carrot, and tomato until the onions are tender; stir frequently. Stir in the pasta, broth, water, tomato sauce, oregano, and bay leaf.

Bring the mixture to boil over high heat; reduce the heat to low. Simmer the soup until the pasta softens (al dente), about 15 to 20 minutes. Salt and pepper the soup according to individual taste. Remove the bay leaf before serving. Serve the hot soup garnished with the parsley or cilantro.

6 servings

	Each serving provides:		
68	Calories	15 g	Carbohydrate
3 g	Protein	29 mg	Sodium
0 g	Fat	0 mg	Cholesterol

Quick and Delicious Light Pasta Sauces

17

Carbonara Sauce

Preparation time: 15 minutes

Bits of ham are key to the success of this light, delicate sauce. Turn your next meal into a tantalizing surprise by saturating your next plateful of warm pasta with a creamy ham sauce. This tempting sauce is a satisfying combination of milk, onions, and ham with a smidgen of Parmesan cheese. For extra punch, add a pinch of cayenne, diced green chiles, nutmeg, or parsley. For fewer calories and less cholesterol, trying using an egg-substitute in place of the whole egg.

1 small yellow onion, finely chopped
1/2 cup finely sliced green onions
1 to 2 cloves garlic, crushed in a garlic press
1/2 cup diced, cooked ham (about 1/4 pound)
4 teaspoons flour
2 cups nonfat milk
1 medium-size egg, lightly beaten
2 tablespoons grated nonfat Parmesan cheese
1 to 2 sprigs fresh thyme
1 to 2 teaspoons crushed fresh marjoram
1 to 2 sprigs fresh celery leaves, minced
Salt and freshly ground pepper

Heat a saucepan over medium-high heat. Sauté the yellow and green onions, garlic, and ham until the onions are tender; stir frequently.

Combine the flour, milk, egg, Parmesan, thyme, marjoram, and celery leaves in a small bowl; mix well. Add the milk mixture to the saucepan; stir constantly until the sauce thickens. Salt and pepper according to individual taste. Remove the thyme before serving.

Makes 3 to 3 1/2 cups

Each 1/4 cup serving provides:

42	Calories	4 g	Carbohydrate
4 g	Protein	39 mg	Sodium
1 g	Fat	24 mg	Cholesterol

18

—⁂—

Spicy Mexican-Style Tomato Sauce

Preparation time: 30 minutes

You will never taste a spicy Mexican-style tomato sauce that isn't enticing, colorful, and wonderfully flavorful. This pungent tomato sauce, laced with a spicy green chile and cilantro, complements your favorite pasta with flair. The natural acids in the tomatoes makes this a sturdy, nutritious sauce. If properly refrigerated, this sauce will store up to two weeks in a tightly sealed container. For a smoother sauce, purée the tomatoes before cooking them. For extra sweet flavor, add puréed bell pepper to the sauce.

6 medium-size ripe tomatoes, blanched or roasted,
    peeled, seeded, and finely chopped
1 small yellow onion, chopped
$1/2$ cup finely sliced green onions
1 to 2 cloves garlic, crushed in a garlic press
$1/8$ to 1 fresh serrano chile, minced (optional, for a
    spicier dish)
1 to 2 teaspoons minced fresh oregano leaves
2 bay leaves
1 to 2 sprigs fresh thyme
1 to 3 sprigs fresh cilantro, minced (optional)
Salt and freshly ground pepper

Heat a large saucepan over medium-high heat. Sauté the tomatoes, yellow and green onions, garlic, and serrano chile until the onions are tender; stir frequently.

Stir in the oregano, bay leaves, thyme, and cilantro; reduce the heat to low. Simmer until the sauce thickens, about 15 minutes. Salt and pepper the sauce according to individual taste. Remove the bay leaves and thyme before serving.

Makes 5 to 5 1/2 cups

Each 1/4 cup serving provides:

17	Calories	4 g	Carbohydrate
1 g	Protein	7 mg	Sodium
0 g	Fat	0 mg	Cholesterol

19

Italian-Style Tomato Sauce

Preparation time: 30 minutes

The popularity of pasta is probably largely due to the sauce served on top of the noodles. Over many generations, the Italians have perfected many favorite tomato sauce recipes with a subtle blend of fresh vegetables and savory herbs. If you like, make this eye-appealing sauce in advance and store it in a tightly sealed container in the refrigerator for later use. For a smoother sauce, purée the tomatoes before cooking them. For a distinctive, nutty flavor, try roasting the garlic and onions before adding them to the sauce. Mushrooms, balsamic vinegar, sun-dried tomatoes, meat, or tomato paste are also popular flavor enhancers.

6 medium-size ripe tomatoes, blanched, peeled, seeded, and finely chopped
1 small yellow onion, finely chopped
⅓ cup finely sliced green onions
2 to 3 cloves garlic, crushed in a garlic press
1 to 2 teaspoons minced fresh oregano leaves
1 to 2 bay leaves
1 to 2 sprigs fresh thyme
1 to 2 teaspoons crushed sage leaves
Salt and freshly ground pepper

Heat a large saucepan over medium-high heat. Sauté the tomatoes, yellow and green onions, and garlic until the onions are tender; stir frequently.

Stir in the oregano, bay leaves, thyme, and sage. Reduce the heat to low. Simmer until the sauce thickens, about 15 minutes. Salt and pepper the sauce according to individual taste. Remove the bay leaves and thyme before serving.

Makes 5 to 5¹/₂ cups

Each ¹/₄ cup serving provides:

11	Calories	3 g	Carbohydrate
1 g	Protein	2 mg	Sodium
0 g	Fat	0 mg	Cholesterol

20

Mushroom Cream Sauce

Preparation time: 15 minutes

If you are in the mood for loads of mushrooms, get ready
for this creamy mushroom sauce, which by the way contains very little fat. If you like, add even more mushrooms.
Prepare your fresh, nutritious ingredients carefully and
serve this rich, luxurious sauce over a plate of your favorite pasta. For an interesting alternative and more
color and flavor, add a dash of paprika, spicy, diced
green chiles, or a few vitamin-rich spinach leaves.

1 small yellow onion, finely chopped
½ cup finely sliced green onions
1 to 2 cloves garlic, crushed in a garlic press
1 cup chopped mushrooms
4 teaspoons flour
2 cups nonfat milk
1 teaspoon soy sauce
1 to 2 sprigs fresh celery leaves, minced
Salt and freshly ground pepper

Heat a saucepan over medium-high heat. Sauté the yellow and green onions, garlic, and mushrooms until the onions are tender; stir frequently.

Combine the flour, milk, soy sauce, and celery leaves in a small bowl; mix well. Add the milk mixture to the saucepan; stir constantly until the sauce thickens. Salt and pepper according to individual taste.

Makes 3 to 3¹/₂ cups

Each ¹/₄ cup serving provides:

24	Calories	4 g	Carbohydrate
2 g	Protein	75 mg	Sodium
0 g	Fat	1 mg	Cholesterol

21

※

Creamy Cucumber Sauce

Preparation time: 15 minutes

This is a fragrant, luscious sauce made with onions, fresh
dill, and cucumbers. Ideal with pasta, you can make this
sauce with little fuss or mess in the kitchen. For an enticing variation, you can add fresh corn, other seasonal vegetables, or extra-virgin olive oil. Make this creamy sauce
and gently toss it with rigate, small penne, or small seashell pasta for a very popular pasta dish. You can also
refrigerate and serve this delightful concoction as a zesty
very low-cal dip.

$^1\!/_2$ cup diced green onions
1 to 2 cloves garlic, crushed in a garlic press
1 small cucumber, diced
2 cups nonfat sour cream
1 to 2 teaspoons minced fresh dill
Salt and freshly ground pepper

Heat a saucepan over medium-high heat. Sauté the green onions, garlic, and cucumber until the onions are tender; stir frequently. Reduce the heat to low. Stir in the sour cream and dill; combine well. Salt and pepper according to individual taste.

Makes 3 cups

Each ¼ cup serving provides:

33	Calories	5 g	Carbohydrate
3 g	Protein	63 mg	Sodium
0 g	Fat	0 mg	Cholesterol

22

Spinach and Mushroom Sauce

Preparation time: 15 minutes

What do you wish for in an especially delicious sauce over your next plate of pasta? Spinach and mushrooms subtly blend to create this light, eye-appealing sauce. For other fun variations, try using carrots, leeks, or zucchini in place of the spinach.

1 small yellow onion, finely chopped
$1/2$ cup finely sliced green onions
1 to 2 cloves garlic, crushed in a garlic press
1 $1/2$ cups chopped mushrooms
1 cup finely chopped spinach
4 teaspoons flour
2 cups nonfat milk
1 to 2 teaspoons minced fresh marjoram leaves, without
     the stems
$1/8$ teaspoon nutmeg
Salt and freshly ground pepper

Heat a saucepan over medium-high heat. Sauté the yellow and green onions, garlic, mushrooms, and spinach until the onions are tender; stir frequently.

Combine the flour, milk, marjoram, and nutmeg in a small bowl; mix well. Add the milk mixture to the saucepan; stir constantly until the sauce thickens. Salt and pepper according to individual taste.

Makes 3 to 3¹/₂ cups

Each ¹/₄ cup serving provides:

27	Calories	4 g	Carbohydrate
2 g	Protein	79 mg	Sodium
0 g	Fat	1 mg	Cholesterol

23

—⚜—

Creamy White Sauce

Preparation time: 15 minutes

This very basic, versatile sauce for pasta offers a smooth
white sheen and light creamy flavor. For interesting
variations, try adding exotic taste pleasers like cilantro,
jalapeño, or serrano chiles with Monterey Jack cheese.
Grated Parmesan cheese, pureéd carrots, and fresh herbs,
like dill, tarragon, and rosemary, are other welcome
additions.

1 small yellow onion, finely chopped
½ cup finely sliced green onions
1 to 2 cloves garlic, crushed in a garlic press
4 teaspoons flour
2 cups nonfat milk
1 to 2 sprigs fresh celery leaves, minced
1 to 2 sprigs fresh thyme
Salt and freshly ground pepper

Heat a saucepan over medium-high heat. Sauté the yellow and green onions and garlic until the onions are tender; stir frequently. Combine the flour, milk, celery leaves, and thyme in a small bowl; mix well. Add the milk mixture to the saucepan; stir constantly until the sauce thickens. Salt and pepper according to individual taste. Remove the thyme before serving.

Makes 3 to 3¹/₂ cups

Each ¹/₄ cup serving provides:

22	Calories	4 g	Carbohydrate
2 g	Protein	25 mg	Sodium
0 g	Fat	1 mg	Cholesterol

24

❧

Chunky Marinara Sauce

Preparation time: 30 minutes

This lightly seasoned tomato sauce simmers well with
a savory array of herbs, ripe tomatoes, and dry white
wine. If you prefer, use the plumper Roma tomatoes for
a thicker sauce. I like to make large quantities of this versatile, flavorful sauce. You can store it in tightly sealed
jars for more than a week. Serve the sauce over any variety of pasta, like spaghetti, rigatoni, or mostaccioli.

6 medium-size ripe tomatoes, blanched or roasted, peeled,
    seeded, and finely chopped
1 small yellow onion, finely chopped
1/2 cup finely sliced green onions
1 to 2 cloves garlic, crushed in a garlic press
1 to 2 teaspoons minced fresh basil leaves
1 to 2 teaspoons minced fresh oregano leaves
1 to 2 teaspoons minced fresh sage leaves
1 to 2 bay leaves
1/2 cup dry white wine
Salt and freshly ground pepper

Heat a large saucepan over medium-high heat. Sauté the tomatoes, yellow and green onions, and garlic until the onions are tender; stir frequently.

Stir in the basil, oregano, sage, bay leaves, and wine; reduce the heat to low. Simmer until the sauce thickens as desired, about 15 to 20 minutes. Salt and pepper the sauce according to individual taste. Remove the bay leaves before serving.

Makes 3 to 3¹/₂ cups

Each ¹/₄ cup serving provides:

23	Calories	4 g	Carbohydrate
1 g	Protein	8 mg	Sodium
0 g	Fat	0 mg	Cholesterol

25

❦

Bolognese Sauce

Preparation time: 45 minutes

If you are looking for a lowfat tomato sauce, try this
delicious Italian-style recipe. It captures the essence of
traditional Italian cooking. The recipe uses a delicious
combination of fresh ripe tomatoes, savory herbs, onions,
and ground beef. Garlic gives this sauce just the right
pungency. For a thicker sauce, add tomato paste or use
plump Roma tomatoes.

No stick cooking spray
½ pound extra-lean ground beef (about 1 cup)
1 small yellow onion, finely chopped
½ cup finely sliced green onions
1 to 3 cloves garlic, crushed in a garlic press
8 medium-size ripe tomatoes, blanched or roasted, peeled,
    seeded, and finely chopped
1 cup chopped mushrooms
1 to 2 teaspoons minced fresh oregano leaves
1 to 2 sprigs fresh thyme
1 to 2 teaspoons minced fresh sage leaves
1 to 2 teaspoons minced fresh basil leaves
2 to 3 bay leaves
Salt and freshly ground pepper

Spray the bottom of a 5-quart pot with the cooking spray so that the ingredients will not stick to the pot. Heat the pot over medium-high heat. Evenly brown the meat, about 5 minutes; stir frequently. Drain the excess fat.

Stir in the yellow and green onions and garlic, tomatoes, and mushrooms. Sauté until the onions are tender. Add the oregano, thyme, sage, basil, and bay leaves; combine well. Bring the sauce to a boil; reduce the heat to low. Simmer the sauce until it thickens, about 20 minutes; stir occasionally. Salt and pepper the sauce according to individual taste. Remove the thyme and bay leaves before serving.

Makes 7 to 7¹/₂ cups

Each ¹/₄ cup serving provides:

30	Calories	9 g	Carbohydrate
8 g	Protein	40 mg	Sodium
6 g	Fat	22 mg	Cholesterol

26

❧

Creamy Shrimp Sauce

Preparation time: 15 minutes

This is a delicious way to capture the luscious flavor of shrimp in a light, creamy sauce. The sauce flavor is a combination of milk, tarragon, and succulent shrimp. Clams, scallops, and mussels are also great substitutes in place of the shrimp. If you like the zingy flavor of lemon with your shrimp, add a grating of lemon rind as garnish to each serving.

1 small yellow onion, finely chopped
½ cup finely sliced green onions
1 to 2 cloves garlic, crushed in a garlic press
⅓ pound (¾ cup) fresh medium-size shrimp, peeled, deveined, cleaned, and coarsely chopped
4 teaspoons flour
2 cups nonfat milk
1 to 2 teaspoons minced fresh tarragon leaves
Salt and freshly ground pepper

Heat a saucepan over medium-high heat. Sauté the yellow and green onions, garlic, and shrimp until the shrimp turns pink; stir occasionally.

Combine the flour, milk, and tarragon in a small bowl; mix well. Add the milk mixture to the saucepan; stir constantly until the sauce thickens. Salt and pepper according to individual taste.

Makes 3 1/2 to 4 cups

Each 1/4 cup serving provides:

31	Calories	3 g	Carbohydrate
4 g	Protein	48 mg	Sodium
0 g	Fat	24 mg	Cholesterol

27

—⚜—

Tuna Sauce

Preparation time: 15 minutes

Fresh tuna is the highlight of this super creamy sauce. If
you prefer, substitute a variety of other firm white fish for
the tuna. Simple and easy to prepare, this versatile sauce
serves well over a variety of differently shaped noodles,
like linguine, mostaccioli, rigatoni, or penne pasta. For a
thicker, richer sauce, try adding ¼ cup nonfat sour cream.

No stick cooking spray
1 small yellow onion, finely chopped
½ cup finely sliced green onions
1 to 2 cloves garlic, crushed in a garlic press
1 cup chopped mushrooms
⅓ cup (about 3 ounces) coarsely chopped, fresh tuna
1 tablespoon flour
1 ½ cups nonfat milk
Salt and freshly ground pepper

Spray the bottom of a medium-size saucepan with cooking spray so that the ingredients will not stick to the pan. Heat the saucepan over medium-high heat. Sauté the yellow and green onions, garlic, mushrooms, and tuna until the tuna cooks thoroughly; stir frequently.

Combine the flour and milk in a small bowl; mix well. Add the milk mixture to the saucepan; stir constantly until the sauce thickens. Salt and pepper according to individual taste.

Makes 3 to 3¹/₂ cups

Each ¹/₄ cup serving provides:

26	Calories	3 g	Carbohydrate
3 g	Protein	22 mg	Sodium
0 g	Fat	4 mg	Cholesterol

28

※

Primavera Sauce

Preparation time: 25 minutes

This delightful recipe combines eggplant, mushrooms,
and bell peppers in a light, spring tomato sauce. Cooks
will savor the subtle flavoring of the fresh herbs and
vegetables. For a richer tomato variation, use sun-dried
tomatoes. For an unusual tropical flavor variation, add
one tablespoon lime juice and 1 tablespoon pineapple
juice to the sauce.

8 medium-size ripe tomatoes, blanched or roasted, peeled,
　　seeded, and finely chopped
1 small yellow onion, finely chopped
½ cup finely sliced green onions
2 to 3 cloves garlic, crushed in a garlic press
1 cup sliced mushrooms
1 small bell pepper, chopped
½ cup chopped eggplant
1 to 3 teaspoons minced fresh oregano leaves
1 to 3 teaspoons minced fresh basil leaves
1 to 3 teaspoons minced fresh sage leaves
Salt and freshly ground pepper
1 to 3 sprigs fresh parsley, minced (optional)

Heat a large saucepan over medium-high heat. Sauté the tomatoes, yellow and green onions, garlic, mushrooms, bell pepper, and eggplant until the bell pepper is crisp-tender; stir frequently.

Stir in the oregano, basil, and sage. Reduce the heat to low. Simmer the sauce for 5 to 10 minutes. Salt and pepper the sauce according to individual taste. Garnish with the parsley.

Makes 8 to 8¹/₂ cups

Each ¹/₄ cup serving provides:

8	Calories	2 g	Carbohydrate
0 g	Protein	3 mg	Sodium
0 g	Fat	0 mg	Cholesterol

29

❦

Monterey Sauce

Preparation time: 15 minutes

This unique sauce is bursting with the delectable flavors
of melted cheese and piquant green chile. It is quite simple
to prepare and accents your favorite pasta with a luscious,
spicy essence. It won't be hard to find a number of perfect
occasions where you can use this zippy sauce over your
favorite pasta.

1 small yellow onion, finely chopped
$^1/_2$ cup finely sliced green onions
1 to 2 cloves garlic, crushed in a garlic press
$^1/_4$ to 1 fresh anaheim or jalepeño chile, seeded, washed,
     and finely chopped (optional, for a spicier dish)
4 teaspoons flour
2 cups nonfat milk
3 tablespoons grated nonfat Monterey Jack cheese
Salt and freshly ground pepper

Heat a saucepan over medium-high heat. Sauté the yellow and green onions, garlic, and chile until the onions are tender; stir frequently.

Combine the flour and milk in a small bowl; mix well. Add the milk mixture to the saucepan; stir constantly until the sauce thickens. Reduce the heat to low. Stir in the cheese; stir until the cheese melts. Salt and pepper according to individual taste.

Makes 3 to 3¹/₂ cups

Each ¹/₄ cup serving provides:

33	Calories	4 g	Carbohydrate
3 g	Protein	190 mg	Sodium
1 g	Fat	13 mg	Cholesterol

30

※

Dijon Sauce

Preparation time: 15 minutes

Packed with the heady flavors of Dijon-style mustard, garlic, and fresh herbs, this tangy, light sauce will add pizazz to your favorite kind of pasta. Combined with vegetables, poultry, meat, or seafood, this creamy sauce guarantees a delightful, tangy surprise for every occasion. For a thicker, richer sauce, try adding 1/4 cup nonfat sour cream. Serve this sauce on ribbon noodles or rigate pasta.

1 small yellow onion, finely chopped
1/2 cup finely sliced green onions
1 to 2 cloves garlic, crushed in a garlic press
4 teaspoons flour
2 cups nonfat milk
1 to 2 tablespoons Dijon-style mustard
1 to 2 teaspoons minced fresh dill
1 to 2 sprigs fresh celery leaves, minced
Salt and freshly ground pepper

Heat a saucepan over medium-high heat. Sauté the yellow and green onions and garlic until the onions are tender; stir frequently.

Combine the flour, milk, mustard, dill, and celery in a small bowl; mix well. Add the milk mixture to the saucepan; stir constantly until the sauce thickens. Salt and pepper according to individual taste.

Makes 3 to 3¹/₂ cups

Each ¹/₄ cup serving provides:

24	Calories	4 g	Carbohydrate
2 g	Protein	55 mg	Sodium
0 g	Fat	1 mg	Cholesterol

31

Tetrazzini Sauce

Preparation time: 15 minutes

This is a smooth, mouth-watering, creamy sauce that goes especially well with vegetables, turkey, and chicken. It serves nicely over many shapes and types of pastas. For additional color and appeal, add peas, broccoli, or carrots to this light, fragrant sauce.

1 small yellow onion, finely chopped
½ cup finely sliced green onions
1 to 2 cloves garlic, crushed in a garlic press
1 bay leaf
1 cup chopped mushrooms
1 cup low-sodium chicken broth
4 teaspoons flour
2 cups nonfat milk
1 tablespoon grated nonfat Parmesan cheese
Salt and freshly ground pepper

Heat a medium-size saucepan over medium-high heat. Sauté the yellow and green onions, garlic, bay leaf, and mushrooms until the onions are tender; stir frequently.

Combine the broth, flour, milk, and Parmesan in a small bowl; mix well. Add the milk mixture to the saucepan; stir constantly until the sauce thickens. Salt and pepper according to individual taste. Remove the bay leaf before serving.

Makes 3 to 3¹/₂ cups

Each ¹/₄ cup serving provides:

25	Calories	4 g	Carbohydrate
2 g	Protein	28 mg	Sodium
0 g	Fat	1 mg	Cholesterol

32

※

Sauce Mornay

Preparation time: 15 minutes

This delectable sauce features the subtle, blended flavors of white wine, onions, and Parmesan cheese. The list of different pastas and ingredients that you can serve with this simple sauce is almost limitless. This sauce also tastes wonderful with extra-lean chicken, turkey, and assorted chunks of seafood. For different variations, add sprigs of dill, rosemary, or parsley.

1 small yellow onion, finely chopped
$^1/_2$ cup finely sliced green onions
1 to 2 cloves garlic, crushed in a garlic press
1 to 2 sprigs fresh thyme
4 teaspoons flour
2 cups nonfat milk
$^1/_4$ cup grated nonfat Parmesan cheese
2 to 3 tablespoons white wine
Salt and freshly ground pepper

Heat a saucepan over medium-high heat. Sauté the yellow and green onions, garlic, and thyme until the onions are tender; stir frequently.

Combine the flour, milk, Parmesan, and wine in a small bowl; mix well. Add the milk mixture to the saucepan; stir constantly until the sauce thickens. Salt and pepper according to individual taste. Remove the thyme before serving.

Makes 3 to 3¹/2 cups

Each ¹/4 cup serving provides:			
26	Calories	4 g	Carbohydrate
2 g	Protein	36 mg	Sodium
0 g	Fat	1 mg	Cholesterol

33

❧

Tuna Garnish

Preparation time: 20 minutes

Dress up your next pasta dish with tuna, chiles, and
tomatoes. Family and friends will especially enjoy this
sumptuous combination served over a warm, fluffy bed of
pasta with a fresh garden salad. For additional appeal, try
adding feta or cottage cheese, minced cilantro, or parsley.

1 teaspoon extra-virgin olive oil
1 small yellow onion, chopped or finely sliced
$^{1}/_{2}$ cup finely sliced green onions
1 to 2 cloves garlic, crushed in a garlic press
$^{1}/_{2}$ cup (about $^{1}/_{4}$ pound) fresh, cleaned tuna chunks
    (1-inch pieces)
1 small ripe tomato, finely chopped
$^{1}/_{4}$ to 1 fresh anaheim or jalapeño chile, seeded, washed,
    and finely chopped (optional, for a spicier dish)
1 to 2 teaspoons minced fresh sage leaves
1 to 2 teaspoons minced fresh marjoram leaves
1 teaspoon Dijon-style mustard
1 tablespoon grated nonfat Monterey Jack cheese
Salt and freshly ground pepper

Heat the oil in a large skillet over medium-high heat. Sauté the yellow and green onions, garlic, tuna, tomato, and chile until the tuna cooks thoroughly; stir frequently. Reduce the heat to low.

Stir in the sage, marjoram, mustard, and cheese; simmer for 2 minutes. Salt and pepper according to individual taste.

Makes 3 to 3¹/₂ cups

	Each serving provides:		
30	Calories	2 g	Carbohydrate
3 g	Protein	32 mg	Sodium
1 g	Fat	6 mg	Cholesterol

34

—❦—

Tomatillo Sauce

Preparation time: 25 minutes

Cooks will love this luscious Southwestern sauce made with little, tart tomatillos. This is a snappy green sauce blended with lime juice, green chile, and tomatoes. To increase the spiciness of the sauce, add more green chile and serve it over penne, rigate, or vermicelli pasta.

1 small yellow onion, finely chopped
1 to 2 cloves garlic, crushed in a garlic press
$\frac{1}{2}$ to 1 fresh anaheim chile, seeded, washed, and finely
    chopped (optional, for a spicier dish)
5 small ripe tomatillos, finely chopped
3 small ripe tomatoes, blanched or roasted, peeled, seeded,
    and finely chopped
$\frac{1}{2}$ cup low-sodium chicken or vegetable broth
2 to 4 sprigs fresh cilantro, minced (optional)
2 to 3 teaspoons lime juice
2 to 3 teaspoons apple cider vinegar
1 to 2 teaspoons minced fresh oregano leaves
Salt and freshly ground pepper

Heat a large saucepan over medium-high heat. Sauté the onion, garlic, anaheim chile, tomatillos, and tomatoes until the onions are tender; stir frequently. Stir in the broth, cilantro, lime juice, vinegar, and oregano; reduce the heat to low. Salt and pepper the sauce according to individual taste. Simmer the sauce until it thickens as desired, about 5 to 10 minutes.

Makes 4 to 4¹/₂ cups

Each ¹/₄ cup serving provides:

12	Calories	3 g	Carbohydrate
1 g	Protein	4 mg	Sodium
0 g	Fat	0 mg	Cholesterol

Light Pasta Dishes with Pizazz

35

—✤—

Scallop Linguine

Preparation time: 20 minutes

If you like to cook with scallops, you will love these
succulent pieces of seafood saturated in a rich, creamy
sauce served over a plateful of warm, chewy pasta. This
linguine recipe is similar to many traditional recipes but
contains less fat. It is also perfect with clams, shrimp, and
other pieces of seafood. For spicier flavor, add a dash of
cayenne pepper, paprika, diced green chiles, or nutmeg.

No stick cooking spray
2 cups (about 4 ounces) dry linguine pasta, cooked ac-
    cording to package directions, drained, and rinsed
1 small yellow onion, chopped
$\frac{1}{2}$ cup finely minced green onions
1 to 2 cloves garlic, crushed in a garlic press
1 cup (about $\frac{1}{2}$ pound) large fresh sea scallops, cleaned in
    cold water
$\frac{1}{2}$ cup finely sliced mushrooms
1 tablespoon flour
1 $\frac{1}{2}$ cups nonfat milk
$\frac{1}{2}$ cup low-sodium broth
$\frac{1}{2}$ teaspoon Worcestershire sauce
1 to 2 sprigs fresh celery leaves, minced
Salt and freshly ground pepper
1 to 3 sprigs fresh parsley, minced (optional)

Spray the bottom of a medium-size saucepan with cooking spray so that the ingredients do not stick to the saucepan. Heat the saucepan over medium-high heat. Sauté the yellow and green onions, garlic, scallops, and mushrooms until the scallops cook thoroughly; stir frequently.

Combine the flour, milk, broth, Worchestershire, and celery in a small bowl; mix well. Add the milk mixture to the saucepan; stir constantly until the sauce thickens. Salt and pepper according to individual taste. Place the warm, cooked linguine on oven-warmed plates. Evenly pour the scallop sauce over the pasta. Sprinkle the dish with the parsley as garnish.

4 servings

Each serving provides:

235	Calories	36 g	Carbohydrate
20 g	Protein	215 mg	Sodium
1 g	Fat	21 mg	Cholesterol

36

Spicy Seafood Creole

Preparation time: 15 minutes
Refrigeration time: 10 to 20 minutes
Cooking time: 10 minutes

This tempting seafood dish offers the exquisitely blended flavors of tomatoes, chiles, and limes. A fresh garden salad and chunk of fresh bread is the perfect accompaniment for this colorful, festive dish. If you like cilantro or parsley, add a few sprigs as garnish. For extra zesty flavor, add wedges of lime.

4 ounces (about 2 cups) dry spaghetti pasta, cooked according to package directions, drained, and rinsed
1/2 cup (about 1/4 pound) fresh fish fillet chunks (1-inch pieces)
1/2 cup (about 1/4 pound) fresh shrimp, peeled, deveined, cleaned, and with the tails removed
1/2 cup (about 1/4 pound) fresh sea scallops, cleaned in cold water
2 tablespoons lime juice
1 teaspoon extra-virgin olive oil
1 small yellow onion, chopped or finely sliced into rings
1/2 cup julienned green onions
1 to 2 cloves garlic, crushed in a garlic press
1/4 to 1 small fresh anaheim chile, diced

¼ cup cooked black beans
2 medium-size ripe tomatoes, finely chopped
½ cup tomato sauce
1 to 2 teaspoons minced fresh basil leaves
1 to 2 sprigs fresh thyme
Salt and freshly ground pepper

Place the seafood pieces and lime juice in a glass baking dish, and toss to thoroughly coat the pieces. Cover; refrigerate the seafood in the marinade for 10 to 20 minutes.

Heat the oil in a large, nonstick skillet over medium-high heat. Sauté the seafood with the marinade, yellow and green onions, garlic, anaheim chile, black beans, and tomatoes, until the onions are tender; stir frequently.

Stir in the tomato sauce, basil, and thyme. Bring to a boil; reduce the heat to low. Simmer the seafood mixture for 10 minutes. Salt and pepper the dish according to individual taste. Remove the thyme before serving. Place the warm, cooked pasta on oven-warmed plates. Pour the seafood sauce over the pasta.

4 servings

Each serving provides:

245	Calories	33 g	Carbohydrate
22 g	Protein	151 mg	Sodium
3 g	Fat	78 mg	Cholesterol

37

Eggplant Primavera

Preparation time: 30 minutes

Here is a deliciously different and healthful way to present an elegant combination of garden fresh vegetables on a soft bed of vermicelli noodles. The eggplant, zucchini, and other vegetables soak in the rich, piquant flavors of herbs and tomatoes. Serve this attractive vermicelli dish as a full satisfying meal or serve smaller portions as an exotic side dish. For a flavorful garnish, sprinkle the pasta dish with nonfat grated Parmesan cheese (about 15 calories per 2 teaspoons).

4 ounces dry vermicelli or rigatoni pasta, cooked
     according to package directions, drained, and rinsed
1 small yellow onion, sliced into rings
$^{1}/_{2}$ small carrot, cut diagonally
1 cup chopped eggplant (1-inch chunks)
1 cup chopped zucchini (1-inch chunks)
1 celery stalk, cut into julienne strips
$^{1}/_{4}$ to 1 small fresh anaheim chile, diced (optional, for
    a spicier dish)
1 teaspoon extra-virgin olive oil
$^{1}/_{2}$ cup finely sliced green onions
1 to 2 cloves garlic, crushed in a garlic press
1 cup small mushroom caps

1 medium-size ripe tomato, finely chopped
1 to 2 teaspoons minced fresh oregano leaves
1 to 2 sprigs fresh celery leaves, minced
Salt and freshly ground pepper

Place a steamer basket inside a 5-quart pot. Bring 1 inch
of water in the pot to the boiling point; reduce the heat to
low. Set the yellow onion, carrot, eggplant, zucchini, celery strips, and anaheim chile into the pot on the steamer
basket. Cook the vegetables, partially covered, until the
vegetables are crisp-tender, about 7 to 9 minutes; drain
the vegetables.
    Heat the oil in a large skillet over medium-high
heat. Sauté the green onions, garlic, mushrooms, tomato,
oregano, and celery leaves until the onions are tender; stir
frequently. Salt and pepper the dish according to individual taste. Place the warm, cooked pasta on oven-warmed
plates. Serve the steamed vegetables over the pasta. Spoon
the tomato sauce over the vegetables and pasta.

4 servings

Each serving provides:

163	Calories	32 g	Carbohydrate
6 g	Protein	33 mg	Sodium
2 g	Fat	0 mg	Cholesterol

38

Shrimp and Pineapples over Vermicelli

Preparation time: 20 minutes

Some ingredients have a delightful way of turning an ordinary dish into a really special meal. Soy sauce and pineapples introduce a distinctive blended flavor in this exotic oriental combination of plump shrimp, pineapple, herbs, and vermicelli pasta. For an attractive, decorative look, butterfly the shrimp and leave the tails on. Spinach linguine or tagliatelle pasta also make an attractive alternative pasta for this dish.

4 ounces dry vermicelli pasta, cooked according to
        package directions, drained, and rinsed
1 small yellow onion, sliced into rings
1/2 cup finely sliced green onions
1 to 2 cloves garlic, crushed in a garlic press
1/2 celery stalk with leaves, diagonally sliced
1/2 small red bell pepper, cut into julienne strips
3/4 pound fresh large shrimp, peeled, deveined, and
        cleaned (about 1 1/2 cups)
1 cup small mushroom caps
1/2 cup chopped pineapple (1-inch chunks)
1/2 cup pineapple juice
2 tablespoons low-sodium soy sauce
Salt and freshly ground pepper

Heat a large, nonstick skillet over medium-high heat. Sauté the yellow and green onions, garlic, celery, bell pepper, shrimp, mushrooms, and pineapple pieces until the shrimp turns pink; stir frequently. Stir in the pineapple juice and soy sauce; reduce the heat to low. Stir in the warm, cooked pasta just before serving; combine well. Salt and pepper the dish according to individual taste.

4 servings

	Each serving provides:		
246	Calories	41 g	Carbohydrate
23 g	Protein	537 mg	Sodium
2 g	Fat	166 mg	Cholesterol

39

—⚬❦⚬—

Vegetables and Pasta

Preparation time: 20 minutes

This is a fragrant, all-veggie meal with beans for additional protein. Serve your pasta dish with a sprinkle of grated nonfat Parmesan or Jack cheese for extra flavor and appeal. If you prefer a pasta dish with a Mediterranean twist, sauté the vegetables in 1 teaspoon extra-virgin olive oil (40 calories per teaspoon).

6 ounces dry vermicelli pasta, cooked according to
    package directions, drained, and rinsed
1 small yellow onion, sliced into rings
½ cup finely sliced green onions
1 to 2 cloves garlic, crushed in a garlic press
6 to 7 fresh broccoli florets, cut in half
½ cup corn kernels
1 cup small mushroom caps
1 small ripe tomato, finely chopped
¼ cup low-sodium vegetable broth
¼ cup cooked garbanzo or red beans
1 to 2 teaspoons minced fresh marjoram or dill
Salt and freshly ground pepper
1 to 3 sprigs fresh parsley, minced (optional)

Heat a large, nonstick skillet over medium-high heat. Sauté the yellow and green onions, garlic, broccoli, corn, mushrooms, and tomato until the broccoli is crisp-tender; stir frequently.

Stir in the broth, beans, and marjoram. Continue to cook for 2 minutes; reduce the heat to low. Stir in the cooked pasta just before serving; combine well. Salt and pepper according to individual taste. Serve the pasta dish on oven-warmed plates. Garnish the dish with the parsley.

4 servings

Each serving provides:

195	Calories	40 g	Carbohydrate
7 g	Protein	38 mg	Sodium
1 g	Fat	0 mg	Cholesterol

40

Creamy Vegetable Pasta Medley

Preparation time: 20 minutes

This vegetable medley overflows with an appealing, creamy sauce. Make your life enjoyable with the succulent flavors and rich colors that are perfect for a nourishing pasta dish. Serving vegetables in a cream sauce is a favorite of most cooks, especially if it is a light, flavorful lowfat sauce.

2 cups (about 4 ounces) dry small ribbon noodles, cooked
    according to package directions, drained, and rinsed
1 small red onion, quartered and separated into sections
7 to 8 fresh cauliflower florets, cut in half
7 to 8 fresh broccoli florets, cut in half
6 to 7 baby carrots, cut in half lengthwise
$^{1}/_{4}$ to 1 small fresh anaheim chile, cut into thin rings
    (optional, for a spicier dish)
1 cup halved fresh mushrooms caps
1 to 2 cloves garlic, crushed in a garlic press
$^{1}/_{4}$ cup sliced green onions
1 tablespoon flour
1 cup nonfat milk
$^{1}/_{2}$ cup nonfat ricotta cheese
1 to 2 teaspoons minced fresh marjoram leaves
Salt and freshly ground pepper

Place a steamer basket inside a 5-quart pot. Bring 1 inch of water in the pot to the boiling point; reduce the heat to low. Set the red onion, cauliflower, broccoli, carrots, and anaheim chile on the steamer basket in the pot. Cook the vegetables, partially covered, about 5 to 6 minutes. Add the mushrooms and cook the vegetables until crisp-tender, about 3 to 4 minutes; drain the vegetables.

Heat a large skillet over medium-high heat. Sauté the garlic and green onions for 1 minute. Combine the flour, milk, ricotta, and marjoram in a small bowl; mix well. Add the milk mixture to the skillet; stir constantly until the sauce thickens. Reduce the heat to low. Toss the steamed vegetables in the creamy sauce. Salt and pepper according to individual taste. Place the warm, cooked pasta on oven-warmed plates. Serve the creamy vegetable sauce over the pasta.

4 servings

Each serving provides:

189	Calories	34 g	Carbohydrate
12 g	Protein	96 mg	Sodium
1 g	Fat	1 mg	Cholesterol

Light Pasta Dishes with Pizazz   95

41

Chile Strips over Pasta

Preparation time: 15 minutes

A simple green chile dish such as this is quite easy to prepare and enjoyed by even your most discriminating diner.
The thin strips of chile, served over ribbon noodles, are
inviting as a unique side dish. Tomatoes provide additional
color and flavor as a bright red garnish over the pasta and
chiles.

2 cups (about 4 ounces) dry ribbon noodles, cooked
    according to package directions, drained, and rinsed
1 teaspoon extra-virgin olive oil
1 small yellow onion, finely sliced into rings
$1/2$ cup finely sliced green onions
1 to 2 cloves garlic, crushed in a garlic press
1 small fresh anaheim chile, cut into thin strips
1 medium-size ripe tomato, finely chopped
1 to 2 teaspoons minced fresh oregano leaves
Salt and freshly ground pepper
2 to 4 sprigs fresh cilantro, minced

Heat the oil in a large, nonstick skillet over medium-high heat. Sauté the yellow and green onions, garlic, chile, tomato, and oregano until the onions are tender; stir frequently. Salt and pepper according to individual taste. Place the warm, cooked pasta on oven-warmed plates. Serve the chile mixture over the pasta. Garnish the dish with the cilantro.

4 servings

140	Calories	27 g	Carbohydrate
5 g	Protein	32 mg	Sodium
2 g	Fat	0 mg	Cholesterol

Each serving provides:

42

—❦—

Penne with Spicy Green Beans and Mushrooms

Preparation time: 20 minutes

This brightly colored vegetable dish is quick and easy to prepare and full of savory flavors. Green bean lovers will appreciate having a lowfat recipe for their favorite green bean dish covered with mushrooms and a thick, creamy sauce.

1 ½ cups (about 3 ounces) dry penne pasta, cooked ac-
    cording to package directions, drained, and rinsed
1 ½ cups diagonally sliced green beans
1 small yellow onion, finely chopped
½ cup finely sliced green onions
1 to 2 cloves garlic, crushed in a garlic press
1 ½ cups finely sliced mushrooms
½ cup nonfat sour cream
¼ cup low-sodium vegetable or chicken broth
1 to 2 teaspoons minced fresh sage leaves
Salt and freshly ground pepper

Heat a large, nonstick skillet over medium-high heat.
Place the green beans with 2 tablespoons of water in the
skillet; cover. Cook until crisp-tender. Stir in the yellow
and green onions, garlic, and mushrooms; sauté until the
onions are tender. Reduce the heat to low.

Stir in the sour cream, broth, and sage; combine well.
Salt and pepper the dish according to individual taste.
Place the warm, cooked pasta on oven-warmed plates.
Serve the green beans and sauce over the pasta.

4 servings

Each serving provides:

138	Calories	27 g	Carbohydrate
7 g	Protein	76 mg	Sodium
1 g	Fat	0 mg	Cholesterol

43

Grilled Vegetable Kabobs over Fideo

Preparation time: 20 minutes
Refrigeration time: 15 minutes
Grilling time: 8 to 10 minutes

Kabob lovers will appreciate this exotic recipe for kabobs
served over a nest of fideo pasta. The fresh basil leaves
sneak in an extra twist of flavor. For a deliciously different
combination, you might like to try using tofu or shrimp in
this recipe. If you cannot grill outdoors, you can also broil
the kabobs four to five inches under the broiler or cook in
a cast iron grill pan.

4 ounces dry fideo pasta, cooked according to package
    directions, drained, and rinsed
1 to 2 cloves garlic, crushed in a garlic press
1 to 2 teaspoons minced fresh basil leaves
1 tablespoon low-sodium soy sauce
1 tablespoon lime juice
¼ cup low-sodium vegetable broth
1 teaspoon extra-virgin olive oil
½ small eggplant, cut into 8 chunks (1 ½ inch wide)
1 small zucchini, cut into 8 chunks (1 ½ inch wide)
4 cherry tomatoes, cut in half
8 small mushrooms caps
8 pineapple chunks (1 ½ inch wide)

1 red bell pepper, cut into 8 chunks (1 1/2-inch wide)
1/3 cup finely sliced green onions
1/4 cup tomato sauce
1 to 2 teaspoons minced fresh oregano leaves
Salt and freshly ground pepper

Combine the garlic, basil, soy sauce, lime juice, broth, and oil in a glass baking dish. Toss the eggplant, zucchini, tomatoes, mushrooms, pineapples, and bell pepper in the marinade to thoroughly coat with the juices. Cover; refrigerate for 15 minutes; turn occasionally. Remove the ingredients from the marinade; reserve the marinade.

Alternately skewer the marinated fruit and vegetables on metal skewers. Grill the kabobs 4 to 5 inches above a bed of hot coals for 4 to 5 minutes on each side.

Heat a large saucepan over medium-high heat. Warm the reserved marinade, green onions, tomato sauce, and oregano. Reduce the heat to low. Stir in the cooked pasta just before serving; combine well. Place the pasta on oven-warmed plates. Lay the skewered kabobs on top of the pasta. Salt and pepper according to individual taste.

4 servings

Each serving provides:

158	Calories	34 g	Carbohydrate
6 g	Protein	167 mg	Sodium
2 g	Fat	0 mg	Cholesterol

44

Spinach and Crumbled Egg Pasta Medley

Preparation time: 20 minutes

If you like spinach, you will love preparing this dramatically different dish. Light texture plus great flavor makes this a perfect dinner entrée or buffet dish. For extra protein, add cooked garbanzo beans. Give your family and friends a taste of this eye-appealing, simple dish and they will request it again and again. For a tasty variation, try adding fresh basil leaves as a scintillating flavor addition.

2 cups (about 4 ounces) dry rigate pasta, cooked according to package directions, drained, and rinsed
1 small yellow onion, chopped
1/2 cup chopped green onions
1 to 2 cloves garlic, crushed in a garlic press
1/2 cup small mushroom caps, stems removed
1/4 bunch (6 ounces) spinach leaves, torn into pieces
(about 2 cups)
1/4 cup grated nonfat Parmesan cheese
Salt and freshly ground pepper
1 hard-cooked egg, diced

Heat a large, nonstick skillet over medium-high heat. Sauté the yellow and green onions, garlic, mushrooms, and spinach with 2 tablespoons water until the onions are tender; stir frequently. Reduce the heat to low.

Stir in the cooked pasta and Parmesan cheese just before serving; combine well. Salt and pepper the sauce according to individual taste. Serve the pasta dish on oven-warmed plates. Garnish the dish with the diced hard-cooked egg.

4 servings

Each serving provides:

152	Calories	28 g	Carbohydrate
9 g	Protein	80 mg	Sodium
2 g	Fat	54 mg	Cholesterol

45

Three Pasta Primavera

Preparation time: 20 minutes

The mouth-watering combination of tomato, corn, and mushrooms dramatically complements any variety of pasta. For additional color, add snappy green beans, garbanzo beans, or eggplant. A fresh garden salad and a chunk of fresh bread are perfect with this nutritious, attractive dish. Garnish with grated nonfat Parmesan cheese (about 15 calories per 2 teaspoons) for extra flavor.

2 cups (about 4 ounces) dry rotelle, mostaccioli, and
    rigatoni pasta, cooked according to package
    directions, drained, and rinsed
1 small yellow onion, chopped
1 to 3 cloves garlic, crushed in a garlic press
½ cup fresh corn kernels, uncooked (about 1 ear)
1 small zucchini, sliced
½ cup small mushroom caps
1 medium-size ripe tomato, finely chopped
1 cup tomato sauce
1 to 2 teaspoons minced fresh oregano leaves
1 to 2 sprigs fresh thyme
Salt and freshly ground pepper

Heat a large, nonstick skillet over medium-high heat. Sauté the onion, garlic, corn, zucchini, mushrooms, and tomato until the zucchini slices are tender; stir frequently. Stir in the tomato sauce, oregano, and thyme; combine well. Reduce the heat to low. Simmer for 5 minutes. Salt and pepper the dish according to individual taste. Remove the thyme before serving. Place the warm, cooked pasta on oven-warmed plates. Serve the sauce over the pasta.

4 servings

Each serving provides:

165	Calories	34 g	Carbohydrate
6 g	Protein	21 mg	Sodium
1 g	Fat	0 mg	Cholesterol

46

—❧—

Curried Mushrooms and Peas over Rigatoni

Preparation time: 20 minutes

A savory blend of mushrooms and peas soaked in a light curry sauce creates a fabulous low-cal pasta dish for special meals with family and friends. Serve over carrot or spinach pasta for additional color and flavor. Sprinkle diced, hard-cooked eggs over the dish for an attractive garnish and added protein.

2 cups (about 4 ounces) dry rigatoni pasta, cooked
     according to package directions, drained, and rinsed
1 small yellow onion, finely sliced
½ cup finely sliced green onions
1 to 2 cloves garlic, crushed in a garlic press
1 ½ cups small mushroom caps
½ cup fresh snow peas or garden peas
2 teaspoons flour
½ cup nonfat milk
½ cup nonfat ricotta cheese
1 teaspoon minced fresh marjoram leaves
¼ to 1 teaspoon curry powder
Salt and freshly ground pepper
2 to 4 sprigs fresh mint leaves (optional)

Heat a large, nonstick skillet over medium-high heat. Sauté the yellow and green onions, garlic, mushrooms, and peas until the peas are crisp-tender; stir frequently. Combine the flour, milk, ricotta, marjoram, and curry powder in a small bowl; mix well. Add the milk mixture to the skillet; stir constantly until the sauce thickens. Reduce the heat to low. Stir in the warm, cooked pasta just before serving; combine well. Salt and pepper the dish according to individual taste. Garnish the dish with the mint leaves.

4 servings

Each serving provides:

154	Calories	26 g	Carbohydrate
10 g	Protein	67 mg	Sodium
1 g	Fat	1 mg	Cholesterol

47

—❧—

Parmesan Mostaccioli and Rotini

Preparation time: 20 minutes

This broccoli dish receives high marks for its nutritious content. Packed with vitamins, potassium, calcium, fiber, and beta-carotene, the ingredients are a tempting combination of vegetables, cheese, and a creamy white sauce. Served in smaller portions as a side dish, this pasta is excellent with a plate of large grilled shrimp or chicken kabobs.

3 cups (about 6 ounces) dry mostaccioli and rotini pasta, cooked according to package directions, drained, and rinsed
1 small yellow onion, chopped
$1/2$ cup sliced green onions (2-inch stalks)
1 to 2 cloves garlic, crushed in a garlic press
7 to 8 fresh broccoli florets, cut into quarters
$1/2$ small zucchini, sliced
$1/2$ cup sliced mushrooms
$3/4$ cup nonfat milk
$1/3$ cup nonfat cream cheese
2 tablespoons grated nonfat Parmesan cheese
1 to 2 teaspoons minced fresh marjoram leaves
Salt and freshly ground pepper
2 to 4 sprigs fresh parsley, minced (optional)

Heat a large, nonstick skillet over medium-high heat. Sauté the yellow and green onions, garlic, broccoli, zucchini, and mushrooms until the zucchini are crisp-tender; stir frequently. Combine the milk, cream cheese, Parmesan, and marjoram in a small bowl; mix well. Add the milk mixture to the skillet; stir constantly until the sauce thickens. Reduce the heat to low.

Stir in the warm, cooked pasta just before serving; combine well. Salt and pepper according to individual taste. Garnish the dish with the parsley.

4 servings

Each serving provides:

219	Calories	41 g	Carbohydrate
14 g	Protein	205 mg	Sodium
1 g	Fat	4 mg	Cholesterol

48

---❦---

Triple Italiano Creole

Preparation time: 20 minutes

In this hearty concoction, the vegetables are cut into small chunks to produce an interesting rough texture. The vegetables simmer gently in a light combination of tomato sauce and herbs. Served over assorted pasta shapes, this dish will delight your diners with an enticing array of flavors, aromas, textures, and colors.

2 cups (about 4 ounces) dry assorted pasta (rotini, mostaccioli, and shells), cooked according to package directions, drained, and rinsed
1 small zucchini, cut into julienne strips
1 cup chopped eggplant (1-inch chunks)
1/2 cup fresh corn kernels, uncooked (about 1 ear)
1 small yellow onion, cut into 1-inch chunks
1/2 cup sliced green onions (2-inch strips)
1/2 small red bell pepper, sliced
1 to 2 cloves garlic, crushed in a garlic press
1 medium-size ripe tomato, finely chopped
1/2 cup low-sodium vegetable broth
1/4 cup tomato sauce
1 to 2 teaspoons minced fresh oregano leaves
1 to 2 teaspoons minced fresh marjoram leaves
Salt and freshly ground pepper
Dash of cayenne pepper (optional, for a spicier dish)

Place a steamer basket inside a 5-quart pot. Bring 1 inch of water in the pot to the boiling point. Reduce the heat to low. Place the zucchini, eggplant, corn, yellow and green onions, and bell pepper into the pot on the steamer basket. Cook the vegetables, partially covered, for 5 to 7 minutes until the zucchini is crisp-tender.

Heat a saucepan over medium-high heat. Warm the garlic, tomato, broth, tomato sauce, oregano, and marjoram. Salt and pepper the dish according to individual taste. Place the warm, cooked pasta on oven-warmed plates. Arrange the steamed vegetables over the pasta. Pour the hot tomato sauce over the vegetables and pasta. Garnish the dish with the cayenne pepper.

4 servings

Each serving provides:

198	Calories	42 g	Carbohydrate
7 g	Protein	23 mg	Sodium
2 g	Fat	0 mg	Cholesterol

49

—❦—

Grilled Halibut Kabobs

Preparation time: 20 minutes
Refrigeration time: 20 minutes
Grilling time: 10 to 14 minutes

The words "fresh" and "zesty" perfectly describe this exquisite, easy-to-prepare kabob dish. The fresh fish pieces literally cook in the juice and absorb the penetrating flavors subtly blended with ginger and soy sauce. Extend your marinade time up to two hours for even more flavor. The hot sizzling apples add sweet taste appeal to the grilled fish. If you prefer, use fresh swordfish instead of halibut in this recipe. If you cannot grill outdoors, you can also broil these pieces of halibut four to five inches under the broiler or cook in a cast iron grill pan.

4 ounces dry angel hair pasta, cooked according to
     package directions, drained, and rinsed
1 pound Halibut, cut into 1 1/2-inch chunks
4 teaspoons apple cider vinegar
2 tablespoons low-sodium soy sauce
2 tablespoons lime juice
1 to 2 teaspoons grated fresh ginger
1 small yellow onion, cut into chunks
1 small apple, cut into 8 chunks
8 small mushrooms caps
1/2 cup sliced pineapple (1-inch chunks)
1/2 cup sliced green onions, (2-inch strips)

1 to 2 cloves garlic, crushed in a garlic press
1 teaspoon extra-virgin olive oil
1 teaspoon water
Salt and freshly ground pepper

Clean the halibut in cold water; pat dry. Combine the vinegar, soy sauce, lime juice, and ginger in a glass baking dish. Toss the halibut, yellow onion, apple, mushrooms, and pineapple in the marinade to thoroughly coat the pieces with the juices. Cover; refrigerate for 20 minutes; turn the pieces occasionally. Remove the pieces from the marinade; reserve the marinade.

Alternately skewer the halibut, yellow onion, apple, mushrooms, and pineapple on the metal skewers. Grill the kabobs four to five inches above a bed of hot coals for 5 to 7 minutes on each side.

Warm the reserved marinade, green onions, garlic, oil, and water in a saucepan over medium-heat; stir occasionally. Reduce the heat to low. Stir in the warm, cooked pasta just before serving; combine well. Salt and pepper the dish according to individual taste. Place the pasta on oven-warmed plates. Lay the kabobs on top of the pasta.

4 servings

Each serving provides:

258	Calories	33 g	Carbohydrate
26 g	Protein	323 mg	Sodium
3 g	Fat	54 mg	Cholesterol

50

—❦—

Grilled Shrimp with Pesto

Preparation time: 30 minutes
Refrigeration time: 15 to 30 minutes
Grilling time: 8 to 10 minutes

This succulent shrimp dish highlights the tasty combination of shrimp and pesto. Quickly grilled over hot coals, you can serve this super easy-to-prepare dish within minutes. If you cannot grill outdoors, you can use metal skewers under the broiler or cook in a cast iron grill pan. A fresh fruit salad will superbly complement this appealing seafood meal. The shrimp are especially attractive if you serve the shrimp butterflied with their tails intact.

4 ounces dry angel hair pasta, cooked according to
    package directions, drained, and rinsed
3 tablespoons lime juice
1 tablespoon water
2 tablespoons apple cider vinegar
1 1/4 pounds fresh jumbo shrimp, peeled, deveined, and
    cleaned (about 2 1/2 cups)
1 teaspoon extra-virgin olive oil
1 small yellow onion, sliced
1/2 cup finely sliced green onions
1 to 2 cloves garlic, crushed in a garlic press
1/2 small red bell pepper, cut into short julienne strips

5 to 10 fresh basil leaves, minced
Salt and freshly ground pepper
2 to 4 sprigs fresh parsley (optional)

Combine the lime juice, water, and apple cider vinegar in a glass baking dish. Toss the shrimp in the marinade to thoroughly coat the shrimp with the juices. Cover; refrigerate the shrimp for 15 to 30 minutes; turn the shrimp pieces occasionally.

Remove the shrimp from the marinade; reserve the marinade. Skewer the shrimp on metal skewers. Grill the shrimp for 4 to 5 minutes on each side until the shrimp turns pink.

Heat the oil in a large skillet over medium-high heat. Sauté the yellow and green onions, garlic, bell pepper, and basil until the bell pepper is tender; stir frequently. Add the reserved marinade. Stir the pasta in the sauce just before serving; combine well. Salt and pepper according to individual taste. Place the warm, cooked pasta on oven-warmed plates. Lay the skewered shrimp over the dish. Garnish the dish with the parsley.

4 servings

	Each serving provides:		
240	Calories	29 g	Carbohydrate
34 g	Protein	242 mg	Sodium
4 g	Fat	228 mg	Cholesterol

51

—❦—

Turkey Rolls and Pasta

Preparation time: 10 minutes
Cooking time: 12 to 15 minutes

Stuffed with mushrooms and herbs, cooks will love these
charming turkey rolls smothered in a rich, savory tomato
sauce. You can speed up cooking time by pre-cooking the
turkey rolls and storing them in a tightly sealed container.

4 ounces dry fettucine pasta, cooked according to package
    directions, drained, and rinsed
³/₄ pound extra-lean ground turkey
1 small yellow onion, finely chopped
¹/₂ cup finely minced green onions
1 to 2 cloves garlic, crushed in a garlic press
¹/₂ cup finely chopped fresh mushrooms
2 teaspoons extra-virgin olive oil
1 cup low-sodium turkey broth
1 medium-size ripe tomato, chopped
1 to 2 teaspoons minced fresh oregano leaves
1 to 2 sprigs fresh thyme
Salt and freshly ground pepper
¹/₂ cup minced fresh parsley (optional)

Combine the turkey, yellow and green onions, garlic, and mushrooms in a medium-size bowl. Shape the turkey mixture into eight individual rolls about 1 inch thick.

Heat the oil in a large skillet over medium-high heat. Cook the turkey rolls until evenly brown, about 7 to 10 minutes; turn occasionally. Add the broth, tomato, oregano, and thyme. Reduce the heat to low. Cover; simmer for 5 minutes. Salt and pepper the dish according to individual taste. Remove the thyme before serving. Place the warm, cooked pasta on oven-warmed plates. Pour the hot tomato sauce and turkey rolls over the pasta. Garnish with the parsley.

4 servings

Each serving provides:

297	Calories	30 g	Carbohydrate
23 g	Protein	103 mg	Sodium
12 g	Fat	75 mg	Cholesterol

52

— ✤ —

Ratatouille Provençale

Preparation time: 25 minutes

The savory combination of onions, tomatoes, eggplant,
and zucchini has long been a popular Italian tradition.
The enticing blend of aromatic herbs, assorted chunks of
vegetables, and spicy, rich red sauce is an elegant, festive
union of brilliant colors and textures. Served over a bed
of vermicelli noodles cooked al dente, this is an incredibly
succulent, fulfilling meal. Use chopped or sliced black
olives as an extra-attractive garnish.

4 ounces dry vermicelli or rigate pasta, cooked according
    to package directions, drained, and rinsed
1 teaspoon extra-virgin olive oil
1 small eggplant, coarsely chopped
1 small zucchini, halved lengthwise and cut into ¹/₂-inch
    slices
1 small yellow onion, finely sliced into rings
¹/₂ cup finely sliced green onions
1 to 2 cloves garlic, crushed in a garlic press
¹/₂ cup finely sliced mushrooms
1 medium-size ripe tomato, coarsely chopped
2 cups tomato sauce
1 to 2 teaspoons minced fresh oregano leaves
1 to 2 teaspoons minced fresh basil leaves
Salt and freshly ground pepper

Heat the oil in a large, nonstick skillet over medium-high heat. Sauté the eggplant and zucchini for 3 minutes. Add the yellow and green onions, garlic, mushrooms, and tomato. Cook until the zucchini is crisp-tender; stir frequently.

Stir in the tomato sauce, oregano, and basil. Reduce the heat to low. Simmer the vegetables in the sauce for 5 minutes. Salt and pepper the dish according to individual taste. Place the warm, cooked pasta on oven-warmed plates. Serve the hot vegetable sauce over the pasta.

4 servings

Each serving provides:

178	Calories	35 g	Carbohydrate
6 g	Protein	27 mg	Sodium
3 g	Fat	0 mg	Cholesterol

53

Seafood Pasta Mornay

Preparation time: 20 minutes

Seafood lovers will enjoy this exotic combination of seafood and vegetables immersed in a creamy white wine sauce. The sauce and variety of fresh, colorful vegetables enhance the exotic, delicate flavor of the seafood. For another smooth variation, you may also want to use octopus, clams, or squid.

2 cups (about 4 ounces) dry rotini and mostaccioli pasta, cooked according to package directions, drained, and rinsed
$^3/_4$ pound (about 1 $^1/_2$ cups) assorted fresh seafood chunks (shrimp, scallops, white fish, or mussels), peeled, deveined, and cleaned in cold water (1-inch pieces)
1 small yellow onion, chopped
$^1/_2$ cup sliced green onions (short julienne strips)
1 to 2 cloves garlic, crushed in a garlic press
1 cup small mushroom caps
6 to 7 fresh cauliflower florets, quartered
4 teaspoons flour
2 cups nonfat milk
$^1/_4$ cup grated nonfat Parmesan cheese

3 tablespoons white wine
1 to 2 sprigs fresh thyme
Salt and freshly ground pepper
1 to 2 sprigs parsley, minced (optional)

Heat a large, nonstick skillet over medium-high heat. Sauté the seafood, yellow and green onions, garlic, mushrooms, and cauliflower until the cauliflower is crisp-tender; stir frequently.

Combine the flour, milk, Parmesan, wine, and thyme in a small bowl; mix well. Add the milk mixture to the skillet; stir constantly until the sauce thickens. Salt and pepper the sauce according to individual taste. Reduce the heat to low. Remove the thyme before serving.

Place the warm, cooked pasta on oven-warmed plates. Serve the hot sauce over the pasta. Garnish the dish with the minced parsley.

4 servings

Each serving provides:

272	Calories	36 g	Carbohydrate
27 g	Protein	263 mg	Sodium
2 g	Fat	80 mg	Cholesterol

54

---&---

Fish Florentine over
Spinach Noodles

Preparation time: 15 minutes
Broiling time: 14 to 18 minutes

Here is an especially quick and simple way to prepare a
light, festive seafood dinner. Combined with interesting
colors and great taste appeal, this recipe subtly blends the
flavors of white fish, mushrooms, and spinach. It is hard
to believe that this dish has so few calories. For a more
formal occasion, serve the fillets and pasta on an oven-
warmed platter.

4 ounces dry spinach noodles, cooked according to pack-
    age directions, drained, and rinsed
4 small firm, white fish fillets, cleaned and skinned
    (about 1 ½ pounds)
1 small yellow onion, chopped
½ cup finely minced green onions
1 to 2 cloves garlic, crushed in a garlic press
½ bunch (about 6 ounces) spinach, coarsely torn into
    pieces (about 2 cups)
½ cup sliced mushrooms
½ cup nonfat sour cream
1 tablespoon grated nonfat Parmesan cheese
Salt and freshly ground pepper

Preheat the broiler. Broil the fish on a baking rack atop a baking sheet on one side for 7 to 9 minutes. Turn the fish over and broil the other side for 7 to 9 minutes. The fish is done when it lightly flakes apart with a fork.

Heat a large, nonstick skillet over medium-high heat. Sauté the yellow and green onions, garlic, spinach, and mushrooms with 2 tablespoons water until the onions are tender; stir frequently. Reduce the heat to low.

Stir in the sour cream and Parmesan; combine well. Salt and pepper according to individual taste. Place the warm, cooked pasta on oven-warmed plates. Lay the cooked fish fillets on the pasta. Pour the hot spinach sauce over the fish and pasta.

4 servings

Each serving provides:

253	Calories	29 g	Carbohydrate
29 g	Protein	215 mg	Sodium
2 g	Fat	54 mg	Cholesterol

55

---&---

Shrimp, Peaches, and Creamy Pasta

Preparation time: 30 minutes

The sophisticated flavors offered by this unique dish will fulfil the dreams of any shrimp lover. The deep, vivid colors of the ripe peaches and bell pepper exquisitely blend with the chewy chunks of shrimp. Served in smaller portions, this is a great starter dish for an elegant seafood dinner. For an interesting variation, you might like to substitute nonfat yogurt in place of the sour cream.

No stick cooking spray
4 ounces dry angel hair pasta, cooked according to
     package directions, drained, and rinsed
1 small yellow onion, chopped
½ cup finely sliced green onion rings
1 celery stalk with leaves, diagonally sliced
1 cup (about ½ pound) fresh medium-size shrimp, peeled,
     deveined, and cleaned
½ small red bell pepper, quartered and cut into
     julienne strips
1 cup (about 2 medium) coarsely chopped peaches
½ cup nonfat sour cream
1 to 2 teaspoons grated fresh ginger
Salt and freshly ground pepper

Spray the bottom of a large, nonstick skillet with cooking spray so that the ingredients do not stick to the skillet. Heat the skillet over medium-high heat. Sauté the yellow and green onions, celery, shrimp, and bell pepper until the shrimp turns pink; stir frequently. Reduce the heat to low.

Stir in the peaches, sour cream, and ginger; combine well. Salt and pepper the dish according to individual taste. Place the warm, cooked pasta on oven-warmed plates. Serve the hot shrimp sauce over the pasta.

4 servings

Each serving provides:

183	Calories	31 g	Carbohydrate
12 g	Protein	130 mg	Sodium
1 g	Fat	35 mg	Cholesterol

56

—❧—

Rotelle with
Mediterranean Scallops

Preparation time: 25 minutes

This seafood dish is an interesting combination of delicate
flavors and exquisite aromas. Served over a bed of pasta
cooked al dente, this is an incredibly flavorful and attractive seafood dish. On more formal occasions, serve this
dish on a platter of wilted spinach leaves garnished with
lots of freshly ground peppercorns and a dash of paprika
or cayenne pepper. It's heavenly!

2 cups (about 4 ounces) dry rotelle or penne pasta, cooked
    according to package directions, drained and rinsed
1 teaspoon extra-virgin olive oil
1 small yellow onion, chopped or finely sliced
1/2 cup finely sliced green onions
1 to 2 cloves garlic, crushed in a garlic press
1 pound fresh sea scallops, cleaned in cold water
    (about 2 cups)
1/2 small green bell pepper, quartered and sliced
1/2 small red bell pepper, quartered and sliced
1/2 cup low-sodium vegetable or fish broth
1 to 2 teaspoons minced fresh basil leaves
1 to 2 sprigs fresh thyme
Salt and freshly ground pepper
1 tablespoon grated nonfat Parmesan cheese

Heat the oil in a large, nonstick skillet over medium-high heat. Sauté the yellow and green onions, garlic, scallops, and bell peppers until the onions are tender; stir frequently. Reduce the heat to low. Stir in the broth, basil, and thyme; combine well.

Simmer the scallop mixture for 5 to 10 minutes; stir occasionally. Salt and pepper the dish according to individual taste. Remove the thyme before serving. Place the warm, cooked pasta on oven-warmed plates. Pour the hot scallop sauce over the pasta. Garnish the dish with the Parmesan cheese.

4 servings

Each serving provides:

238	Calories	30 g	Carbohydrate
24 g	Protein	320 mg	Sodium
3 g	Fat	38 mg	Cholesterol

57

—❦—

Spicy Rainbow Seafood Stew

Preparation time: 10 minutes
Cooking time: 15 to 20 minutes

The sophisticated flavors in this thick, well-seasoned stew will stimulate and satisfy even the most demanding appetite. The deep, vivid colors and chunks of seafood blend well with the aromatic Italian flavors of fresh herbs and tomatoes. Rigate pasta and a sprinkling of Parmesan cheese add irresistible color and texture.

1 teaspoon extra-virgin olive oil
1 yellow onion, finely chopped
1/2 cup finely sliced green onions
1 to 4 cloves garlic, crushed in a garlic press
1/2 cup sliced fresh mushrooms
3/4 pound (about 1 1/2 cups) assorted fresh seafood chunks
    (scallops, shrimp, white fish, clams, or mussels),
    cleaned in cold water (1-inch pieces)
3 ounces (about 1 1/2 cups) dry rigate pasta, uncooked
2 large ripe tomatoes, finely chopped
1/2 small red bell pepper, chopped
1 cup water
1 1/2 cups low-sodium vegetable or fish broth
2 teaspoons lime juice
1 to 2 teaspoons minced fresh oregano leaves
Salt and freshly ground pepper
2 tablespoons grated nonfat Parmesan cheese

Heat the oil in a large soup pot. Sauté the yellow and green onions, garlic, mushrooms, seafood, pasta, tomatoes, and bell pepper until the onions are tender; stir frequently.

Stir in the water, broth, lime juice, and oregano; combine well. Bring the liquid to a boil; reduce the heat to low. Simmer the stew for 15 to 20 minutes. Salt and pepper the dish according to individual taste. Serve the hot steaming stew in bowls garnished with Parmesan cheese.

4 servings

Each serving provides:			
195	Calories	25 g	Carbohydrate
21 g	Protein	183 mg	Sodium
2 g	Fat	78 mg	Cholesterol

58

—✦—

Seafood with Steamed Vegetables

Preparation time: 25 minutes

The seafood and vegetables taste as good as they look. The luscious flavors of these colorful steamed vegetables are perfect for a one-dish meal served over mostaccioli pasta. Vegetable lovers will especially enjoy this tempting feast with a sprinkling of Parmesan cheese. For a formal setting, place the pasta in the middle of a platter surrounded by the steamed vegetables.

2 cups (about 4 ounces) dry mostaccioli pasta, cooked
    according to package directions, rinsed, and drained
1 small yellow onion, quartered and separated into
    sections
10 to 12 fresh cauliflower florets
6 to 7 fresh broccoli florets
1/2 cup thinly sliced red bell pepper rings
1 cup halved fresh mushrooms caps
1/4 pound large fresh sea scallops, cleaned in cold water
    (about 1/2 cup)
1/4 pound large fresh shrimp, peeled, deveined, and
    cleaned (about 1/2 cup)
2 teaspoons extra-virgin olive oil
1/2 cup finely sliced green onions
1 to 2 cloves garlic, crushed in a garlic press

1 to 2 teaspoons minced fresh sage leaves
Salt and freshly ground pepper
2 tablespoons grated nonfat Parmesan cheese

Place a steamer basket inside a 5-quart pot. Bring 1 inch of water in the pot to the boiling point; reduce the heat to low. Set the onion, cauliflower, broccoli, and bell pepper on the steamer basket in the pot. Cook the vegetables, partially covered, about 5 to 7 minutes. Add the mushrooms and seafood; steam until the broccoli is tender and the shrimp turns pink, about 3 to 4 minutes. Drain the vegetables.

Heat the oil in a large, nonstick skillet over medium-high heat. Sauté the green onions, garlic, and sage for 1 minute. Reduce the heat to low. Stir in the cooked pasta just before serving; combine well. Place the pasta on oven-warmed plates. Serve the steamed vegetables over the pasta. Salt and pepper the dish according to individual taste. Garnish with the Parmesan cheese.

4 servings

Each serving provides:

221	Calories	31 g	Carbohydrate
17 g	Protein	168 mg	Sodium
4 g	Fat	65 mg	Cholesterol

59

—❧—

Baked Parmesan Fish

Preparation time: 15 minutes
Baking time: 20 minutes
Preheat oven to 350°

This appetizing fish recipe features white fish fillets coated
with Parmesan cheese. You can easily adapt this unique
baked fish recipe to include most firm, white fish fillets,
including swordfish, sole, halibut, or red snapper. Serve
this delectable, high-protein dish with a side of vegetables
and a fresh fruit salad for dessert

4 ounces dry angel hair pasta, cooked according to
    package directions, drained, and rinsed
¹/₃ cup grated nonfat Parmesan cheese
1 teaspoon flour
2 to 3 sprigs fresh thyme, crushed without the stems
4 small firm, white fish fillets, cleaned and skinned
    (about 1 ¹/₂ pounds)
1 small yellow onion, chopped or finely sliced
¹/₂ cup finely sliced green onions
1 to 2 cloves garlic, crushed in a garlic press
1 cup halved fresh small mushrooms caps
Salt and freshly ground pepper

Place the Parmesan cheese, flour, and thyme in a paper bag. Individually coat the fish by gently shaking the fillets in the bag; reserve the coating ingredients in the paper bag. Bake the fish fillets on a baking rack at 350° for 20 minutes. The fish fillets are done when they flake apart with a fork.

Heat a large, nonstick skillet over medium-high heat. Sauté the yellow and green onions, garlic, and mushrooms until the onions are tender; stir frequently. Salt and pepper according to individual taste. Place the warm, cooked pasta on oven-warmed plates. Attractively arrange the fish fillets on the pasta. Serve the hot mushroom sauce over the fish and pasta. Garnish the dish with the reserved coating ingredients from the paper bag.

4 servings

Each serving provides:

293	Calories	29 g	Carbohydrate
40 g	Protein	216 mg	Sodium
3 g	Fat	81 mg	Cholesterol

60

❦

Spicy Scallops and Pasta

Preparation time: 15 minutes
Cooking time: 10 minutes

Why serve another ordinary meal when you can create a
sensation with this savory, eye-appealing meal of scallops
slowly simmered in a thick, spicy red sauce? Fresh, firm,
large sea scallops combine with soft, warm pasta to create
the perfect light meal. If you want to add an even spicier
twist, try minced cilantro or diced chiles for extra flavor.

4 ounces dry angel hair pasta, cooked according to
      package directions, drained, and rinsed
1 small yellow onion, chopped
1/2 cup finely sliced green onions
1 to 2 cloves garlic, crushed in a garlic press
1/2 small green bell pepper, quartered and thinly sliced
3/4 pound large fresh sea scallops, cleaned in cold water
      (about 1 1/2 cups)
1 cup sliced fresh mushrooms
1 1/2 cups tomato sauce
2 tablespoons red wine (optional)
1 to 2 teaspoons minced fresh oregano leaves
1 to 2 sprigs fresh thyme, crushed without the stem
1 to 2 teaspoons minced fresh marjoram leaves
Salt and freshly ground pepper

Heat a large, nonstick skillet over medium-high heat. Sauté the yellow and green onions, garlic, bell pepper, scallops, and mushrooms until the bell pepper is crisp-tender; stir frequently.

Stir in the tomato sauce, wine, oregano, thyme, and marjoram. Reduce the heat to low. Simmer the dish for 10 minutes; stir occasionally. Salt and pepper the dish according to individual taste. Remove the thyme. Place the warm, cooked pasta on oven-warmed plates. Pour the scallop sauce over the pasta.

4 servings

Each serving provides:

234	Calories	34 g	Carbohydrate
20 g	Protein	157 mg	Sodium
2 g	Fat	29 mg	Cholesterol

61

—✤—

Shrimp and Broccoli Alfredo

Preparation time: 20 minutes

This festive, enticing feast is a colorful array of flavorful, nutritious ingredients. Served over a nest of pasta, the combination of shrimp and broccoli create a delicate, refreshing feast. Scallops, increasingly popular in the United States, are a wonderful substitute for the shrimp in this exquisite dish.

4 ounces dry linguine pasta, cooked according to package
   directions, drained, and rinsed
1 small yellow onion, chopped
½ cup finely minced green onions
1 to 2 cloves garlic, crushed in a garlic press
¾ pound fresh large shrimp, peeled, deveined, and
   cleaned (about 1 ½ cups)
4 to 5 fresh broccoli florets, quartered
4 large fresh mushroom caps, sliced
1 cup nonfat sour cream
¼ cup grated nonfat Parmesan cheese
Salt and freshly ground pepper
4 sprigs fresh rosemary (optional)

Heat a large, nonstick skillet over medium-high heat. Sauté the yellow and green onions, garlic, shrimp, broccoli, and mushrooms until the shrimp turns pink; stir frequently. Reduce the heat to low.

Stir in the sour cream and Parmesan cheese; combine well. Salt and pepper the dish according to individual taste. Place the warm, cooked pasta on oven-warmed plates. Pour the hot shrimp sauce over the pasta. Garnish each dish with a sprig of fresh rosemary.

4 servings

Each serving provides:

256	Calories	33 g	Carbohydrate
28 g	Protein	326 mg	Sodium
2 g	Fat	166 mg	Cholesterol

62

Salmon Steaks in Dijon Sauce

Preparation time: 10 minutes
Refrigeration time: 15 to 30 minutes
Broiling time: 8 to 10 minutes

Soak these elegant salmon steaks in lemon juice, broil
them, and finally, serve them with a light, creamy Dijon-
style sauce over angel hair pasta. The additional flavoring
of tarragon adds the final, delicate touch. You'll want to
try this enticing recipe with other types of firm fish like
halibut or swordfish. A tossed green salad and crusty
piece of Italian bread superbly complement this wonderfully delicious, nutritious meal.

3 ounces dry angel hair pasta, cooked according to
    package directions, drained, and rinsed
4 small fresh pink salmon steaks, deboned and skinned
    (about 1 ½ pounds)
2 tablespoons lemon juice
1 small yellow onion, finely sliced
½ cup sliced green onions
1 to 2 cloves garlic, crushed in a garlic press
⅓ cup nonfat sour cream
1 to 2 teaspoons Dijon-style mustard
1 to 2 teaspoons minced fresh tarragon leaves
Salt and freshly ground pepper
1 to 3 sprigs fresh parsley, minced (optional)

Clean the salmon steaks in cold water; pat dry. Lightly prick both sides of the salmon steaks with a fork. Place the salmon and lemon juice in a glass baking dish. Rub the steaks in the lemon juice to coat the steaks with the juices. Cover; refrigerate the salmon steaks for 15 to 30 minutes; turn the steaks occasionally. Reserve the marinade.

Turn on the broiler. Place the salmon steaks on a broiler rack atop a baking sheet and brush with the reserved marinade. Broil the salmon steaks two to four inches below the heat for 4 to 5 minutes. Turn the salmon steaks over and brush them with the marinade. Continue cooking the salmon steaks under the broiler until the salmon cooks thoroughly, about 4 to 5 minutes. The salmon steaks are done when the flesh easily flakes apart with a fork.

Heat a large nonstick saucepan over medium-high heat. Sauté the yellow and green onions and garlic until the onions are tender; stir frequently. Reduce the heat to low.

Stir in the sour cream, mustard, and tarragon; combine well. Stir in the cooked pasta just before serving; combine well. Place the creamy pasta on oven-warmed plates. Attractively arrange a broiled salmon steak on each plate. Salt and pepper the dish according to individual taste. Garnish the dish with the parsley.

4 servings

Each serving provides:

300	Calories	20 g	Carbohydrate
39 g	Protein	206 mg	Sodium
6 g	Fat	89 mg	Cholesterol

63

—⚘—

Baked Red Snapper over Spaghetti

Preparation time: 10 minutes
Baking time: 20 minutes
Preheat oven to 350°

Choose this recipe for a deliciously different and healthful
way to prepare fresh red snapper. This simple recipe also
works well with any other firm white fish. Fish lovers will
enjoy the subtle blend of lemon juice, Parmesan cheese,
and thyme served over succulent snapper fillets.

No stick cooking spray
3 ounces dry thin spaghetti pasta, cooked according to
        package directions, drained, and rinsed
4 red snapper fillets, cleaned and skinned
        (about 1 ½ pounds)
2 tablespoons grated nonfat Parmesan cheese
1 to 3 sprigs fresh thyme, crushed without the stem
1 to 3 sprigs fresh celery leaves, minced
1 cup fresh small mushroom caps
1 small yellow onion, chopped
½ cup chopped green onions
¼ small fresh anaheim chile, finely chopped
1 to 2 cloves garlic, crushed in a garlic press
1 tablespoon lemon juice
Salt and freshly ground pepper

Spray a large, rectangular glass baking dish with the cooking spray. Place the fillets in the baking dish. Evenly sprinkle the Parmesan cheese, thyme, and celery leaves over the fish.

Combine the mushrooms, yellow and green onions, chile, garlic, and lemon juice in a small bowl; mix well. Evenly spread the ingredients over the fish. Bake the fish in a preheated oven at 350° for 20 minutes. The fish is done when it flakes apart with a fork. Place the warm, cooked pasta on oven-warmed plates. Serve the fish fillets over the warm pasta. Salt and pepper according to individual taste.

4 servings

Each serving provides:

288	Calories	28 g	Carbohydrate
38 g	Protein	165 mg	Sodium
3 g	Fat	81 mg	Cholesterol

Now You're Cooking Main Pasta Dishes

64

~❦~

Mediterranean Grilled
Beef Chunks

Preparation time: 15 minutes
Refrigeration time: 15 minutes
Grilling time: 8 to 10 minutes

This is a recipe for marinated beef chunks, pasta, and
vegetables served with a light tomato sauce. The balsamic
vinegar gives this dish an especially tempting flavor. If you
cannot grill outdoors, you can also broil these chunks of
beef four to five inches under the broiler or cook them in a
cast iron grill pan.

4 ounces dry angel hair or linguine pasta, cooked accord-
     ing to package directions, drained, and rinsed
3 tablespoons lime juice
1 tablespoon balsamic vinegar
³/4 pound extra-lean round steak, cut across the grain into
     1 ¹/2-inch chunks (about 1 ¹/2 cups)
1 teaspoon extra-virgin olive oil
1 small yellow onion, quartered and sliced
¹/2 cup julienned green onions
1 to 2 cloves garlic, crushed in a garlic press
¹/2 small zucchini, sliced
¹/2 small green bell pepper, finely sliced
¹/2 small red bell pepper, finely sliced
1 small ripe tomato, chopped
Salt and freshly ground pepper

Combine the lime juice and vinegar in a glass baking dish. Toss the beef in the marinade to thoroughly coat the beef with the juices. Cover; refrigerate the beef for at least 15 minutes; turn the beef pieces occasionally.

Remove the beef from the marinade. Skewer the beef on metal skewers. Grill the beef four to five inches above a bed of hot coals for 4 to 5 minutes on each side. Cook until the beef is done according to taste.

Heat the oil in a large, nonstick skillet over medium-high heat. Stir in the yellow and green onions, garlic, zuchinni, bell peppers, and tomato. Sauté until the zucchini is tender; stir frequently. Stir in the cooked pasta just before serving; combine well. Salt and pepper according to individual taste. Place the pasta and vegetables on oven-warmed plates. Attractively arrange the chunks of beef on top of the pasta. Serve the hot dish immediately.

4 servings

Each serving provides:

284	Calories	28 g	Carbohydrate
30 g	Protein	66 mg	Sodium
6 g	Fat	59 mg	Cholesterol

65

— ✿ —

Spiced Chicken and Peppers

Preparation time: 20 minutes

The spiced chicken and pasta found in this dish will get
top marks for their special flavor. The spicy anaheim chile
and bell pepper add contrasting color and a distinctive
Latin accent. In the summertime, you can blacken the
chicken on the grill for even more delicious flavor and
eye appeal.

No stick cooking spray
4 ounces dry angel hair pasta, cooked according to
    package directions, drained, and rinsed
¾ pound extra-lean chicken, skinned, boned, and cut into
    tenderloin pieces (about 1½ cups)
1 small yellow onion, sliced into rings
½ cup finely sliced green onions
1 to 2 cloves garlic, crushed in a garlic press
1 celery stalk with leaves, sliced
¼ to 1 small fresh anaheim chile, washed, seeded,
    and diced
½ small green bell pepper, cut into julienne strips
1 medium-size ripe tomato, chopped
½ cup low-sodium chicken broth
½ cup tomato sauce
1 to 2 teaspoons minced fresh oregano leaves
Dash of cayenne pepper (optional, for a spicier dish)
Salt and freshly ground pepper

Spray the bottom of a large, nonstick skillet with the cooking spray so that the ingredients will not stick to the skillet. Heat the skillet over medium-high heat. Evenly brown the chicken to lock in the juices; cook until golden brown, about 3 to 5 minutes per side.

Add the yellow and green onions, garlic, celery, anaheim chile, bell pepper, and tomato; stir frequently until the bell pepper is tender. Stir in the broth, tomato sauce, oregano, and cayenne; stir for 2 minutes. The chicken is done when it pulls apart with a fork. Salt and pepper the dish according to individual taste. Place the warm, cooked pasta on oven-warmed plates. Serve the hot chicken sauce over the pasta.

4 servings

Each serving provides:

263	Calories	54 g	Carbohydrate
37 g	Protein	93 mg	Sodium
3 g	Fat	72 mg	Cholesterol

66

❧

Mandarin Chicken

Preparation time: 20 minutes

A dash of soy sauce and a hint of fresh ginger provide subtle, fragrant flavors to this chicken and pasta dish. For
other enticing variations, you may like to substitute strips
of pork loin or beef in place of the chicken. Served with a
unique combination of broccoli, oranges, and red onions,
this dish displays wonderfully contrasting colors and
scintillating flavors.

No stick cooking spray
4 ounces dry thin spaghetti, cooked according to package
    directions, drained, and rinsed
1 pound extra-lean chicken, skinned, boned, and cut into
    large tenderloin pieces (about 2 cups)
1 small red onion, chopped
1 to 2 cloves garlic, crushed in a garlic press
5 fresh broccoli florets, quartered
$^{1}/_{2}$ cup sliced fresh mushrooms
$^{1}/_{2}$ cup fresh bamboo sprouts
$^{1}/_{2}$ cup mandarin oranges or tangerine slices
2 tablespoons low-sodium chicken broth
2 tablespoons water
2 teaspoons lime juice
$^{1}/_{4}$ cup low-sodium soy sauce
$^{1}/_{2}$ to 1 teaspoon grated fresh ginger
Salt and freshly ground pepper
Dash of paprika or cayenne pepper

Spray the bottom of a large, nonstick skillet with the cooking spray so that the ingredients will not stick to the skillet. Heat the skillet over medium-high heat. Evenly brown the chicken to lock in the juices; cook until golden brown, about 3 to 5 minutes per side.

Stir in the red onion, garlic, and broccoli; stir occasionally until the broccoli is crisp-tender. Add the mushrooms, bamboo sprouts, and orange slices; stir for 2 minutes. Combine the broth, water, lime juice, soy sauce, and ginger in a small bowl; mix well. Stir the soy sauce mixture into the skillet; combine well. Reduce the heat to low.

Simmer the chicken for 5 minutes. The chicken is done when it pulls apart with a fork. Place the warm, cooked pasta on oven-warmed plates. Serve the hot chicken sauce over the pasta. Salt and pepper according to individual taste. Garnish the dish with the paprika or cayenne.

4 servings

Each serving provides:

297	Calories	65 g	Carbohydrate
48 g	Protein	701 mg	Sodium
4 g	Fat	96 mg	Cholesterol

67

---❦---

Fettucine Carbonara

Preparation time: 20 minutes

This traditional Italian dish is simple to prepare and creates a tempting showpiece for a healthful, satisfying meal. Try this light creamy sauce packed with chunks of ham on your next plateful of warm, sweet-smelling pasta. If you prefer, slightly change the recipe by using any left-over chunks of beef, poultry, or seafood.

6 ounces dry fettucine pasta, cooked according to package
    directions, drained, and rinsed
1 small yellow onion, chopped
½ cup finely minced green onions
1 to 3 cloves garlic, crushed in a garlic press
½ pound diced, cooked, extra-lean ham (about 1 cup)
4 teaspoons flour
2 cups milk
1 to 2 tablespoons grated nonfat Parmesan cheese
1 to 2 teaspoons minced fresh celery leaves
Salt and freshly ground pepper
1 to 3 sprigs parsley, minced (optional)

Heat a medium-size saucepan over medium-high heat. Sauté the yellow and green onions, garlic, and ham until the onions are tender; stir frequently. Combine the flour, milk, Parmesan, and celery leaves in a small bowl; mix well. Stir the milk mixture into the saucepan; stir constantly until the sauce thickens. Salt and pepper the sauce according to individual taste.

Place the warm, cooked pasta on oven-warmed plates. Serve the hot ham sauce over the pasta. Garnish the dish with the parsley.

4 servings

Each serving provides:

277	Calories	43 g	Carbohydrate
18 g	Protein	511 mg	Sodium
3 g	Fat	21 mg	Cholesterol

68

Pasta Bows with Beef

Preparation time: 25 minutes

This special dish gets its visual appeal from the pasta bows soaked with tenderized chunks of beef in a rich, hearty tomato sauce. The unique flavor of eggplant blends with the earthy appeal of fresh tomatoes and herbs. In this recipe you will find few calories, colorful ingredients, and lots of hearty Italian-style flavor. Try a dash of nonfat Parmesan cheese as garnish. For extra flavor and a few more calories, sauté the beef in extra-virgin olive oil (about 40 calories per teaspoon).

No stick cooking spray
2 cups (about 4 ounces) dry bow tie pasta, cooked according to package directions, drained, and rinsed
$3/4$ pound extra-lean round steak, cut into $1\frac{1}{2}$-inch medallions (about $1\frac{1}{2}$ cups)
1 small yellow onion, chopped
$\frac{1}{2}$ cup finely minced green onions
1 to 2 cloves garlic, crushed in a garlic press
$\frac{1}{2}$ cup julienned eggplant
$\frac{1}{2}$ cup sliced fresh mushrooms
1 small tomato, finely chopped
$1\frac{1}{2}$ cups tomato sauce
2 to 3 sprigs fresh thyme, crushed without the stem

1 to 2 teaspoons minced fresh marjoram leaves
1 to 2 teaspoons minced fresh oregano leaves
Salt and freshly ground pepper
Dash of cayenne pepper (optional, for a spicier dish)
2 to 4 sprigs fresh parsley, minced (optional)

Spray the bottom of a large, nonstick skillet with the cooking spray so that the ingredients will not stick to the skillet. Heat the skillet over medium-high heat. Evenly brown the beef for 5 minutes; stir frequently. Drain any excess fat.

Stir in the yellow and green onions, garlic, eggplant, mushrooms, and tomato; sauté until the onions are tender. Stir in the tomato sauce, thyme, marjoram, and oregano; reduce the heat to low. Simmer for 3 to 5 minutes. Salt and pepper according to taste. Place the warm, cooked pasta on oven-warmed plates. Pour the hot beef sauce over the pasta. Garnish the dish with cayenne pepper and parsley.

4 servings

Each serving provides:

296	Calories	32 g	Carbohydrate
31 g	Protein	75 mg	Sodium
5 g	Fat	59 mg	Cholesterol

69

Spicy Mexican-Style Steak

Preparation time: 15 minutes
Refrigeration time: 30 minutes
Grilling time: 8 to 10 minutes

Steaks are especially attractive and appetizing when they
are served on a bed of thin noodles soaked in a spicy tomato
sauce. If you prefer a spicier dish, you can add diced anaheim,
jalapeño, or serrano chiles to the dish. If you cannot grill
outdoors, you can also broil the steaks four to five inches
under the broiler or cook in a cast iron grill pan.

No stick cooking spray
2 ounces dry angel hair pasta, cooked according to
     package directions, drained, and rinsed
$^{1}/_{3}$ cup lime juice
4 small, thin extra-lean round or flank steaks
     (about 1 pound)
1 small yellow onion, sliced
$^{1}/_{2}$ cup finely sliced green onions
1 to 2 cloves garlic, crushed in a garlic press
1 medium-size tomato, blanched or roasted, peeled,
     seeded, and finely chopped
$^{1}/_{4}$ to 1 small fresh anaheim chile, seeded, washed, and
     finely chopped (optional, for a spicier dish)
$^{1}/_{2}$ cup tomato sauce
1 to 2 teaspoons minced fresh oregano leaves
Salt and freshly ground pepper
2 to 4 sprigs fresh cilantro, minced (optional)

Place the lime juice and steaks in a glass baking dish. Toss the steaks in the marinade to coat the steaks with the juices. Cover; marinate the steaks in the refrigerator for 30 minutes; turn the steaks occasionally.

Spray the bottom of a large, nonstick skillet with the cooking spray so that the ingredients will not stick to the skillet. Heat the skillet over medium-high heat. Sauté the yellow and green onions, garlic, tomato, and anaheim chile until the onions are tender; stir frequently. Add the tomato sauce and oregano; reduce the heat to low. Simmer the sauce for 5 minutes.

Remove the steaks from the marinade; drain the marinade. Place the steaks four or five inches above a bed of hot coals. Sear both sides of each steak for 1 minute. Grill the steaks for 4 to 5 minutes on each side. Cook the meat according to individual taste.

Stir the warm, cooked pasta into the sauce just before serving. Salt and pepper according to individual taste. Place the pasta on oven-warmed plates. Attractively arrange the grilled steaks on the pasta. Garnish the dish with the cilantro.

4 servings

Each serving provides:			
277	Calories	18 g	Carbohydrate
37 g	Protein	90 mg	Sodium
6 g	Fat	79 mg	Cholesterol

70

—⚜—

Marengo-Style Chicken

Preparation time: 20 minutes
Cooking time: 40 to 45 minutes

Sit down and eat your next family dinner with this great
tasting chicken and pasta dish. It combines the delicious
flavors of white wine, mushrooms, and tomatoes with
juicy breasts of chicken. For an added attraction, garnish
this easy-to-prepare chicken creation with sprigs of fresh
parsley, cilantro, or rosemary.

No stick cooking spray
1 ½ cups (about 3 ounces) dry ribbon noodles, cooked
    according to package directions, drained, and rinsed
1 pound extra-lean chicken breasts, skinned and boned
    (about 4 breast pieces)
1 small yellow onion, sliced
½ cup finely minced green onions
1 to 2 cloves garlic, crushed in a garlic press
1 ½ cups small mushroom caps
3 small ripe tomatoes, finely chopped
1 tablespoon flour
½ cup low-sodium chicken broth
½ cup tomato sauce
⅓ cup dry white wine
1 bay leaf
1 to 2 teaspoons minced oregano leaves
2 to 3 sprigs fresh thyme, crushed without the stem

Salt and freshly ground pepper
4 sprigs fresh rosemary (optional)

Spray the bottom of a large, nonstick skillet with the cooking spray so that the ingredients will not stick to the skillet. Heat the skillet over medium-high heat. Evenly brown the chicken breasts to lock in the juices; cook until golden brown, about 3 to 5 minutes per side. Remove the chicken breasts.

Sauté the yellow and green onions, garlic, mushrooms, and tomatoes in the skillet until the onions are tender; stir occasionally. Combine the flour, broth, tomato sauce, wine, bay leaf, oregano, and thyme in a small bowl; mix well. Stir the wine sauce into the skillet; combine well. Reduce the heat to low.

Place the chicken in the skillet. Cover; simmer for 40 to 45 minutes. The chicken is done when it pulls apart with a fork. If the sauce cooks away, add additional broth, tomato sauce, and wine. Salt and pepper the chicken dish according to individual taste. Remove the bay leaf. Place the pasta on oven-warmed plates. Place the chicken on the pasta. Serve the hot sauce over the chicken. Garnish the dish with the sprigs of rosemary.

4 servings

Each serving provides:

296	Calories	59 g	Carbohydrate
47 g	Protein	103 mg	Sodium
4 g	Fat	96 mg	Cholesterol

71

—❦—

Pork Loin Oriental

Preparation time: 25 minutes

Pork has a high vitamin B content and is an excellent
source of protein and iron. This nutritious pasta dish
has a sparkling, sweet-tart taste from extra-enticing Asian
flavors. For a meatless dish, use tofu as an excellent substitute for the pork in this recipe.

No stick cooking spray
4 ounces dry angel hair pasta, cooked according to
     package directions, drained, and rinsed
³/₄ pound extra-lean pork loin, cut into ¹/₂-inch strips
     (about 1¹/₂ cups)
1 small yellow onion, chopped
¹/₂ cup finely minced green onions
1 to 2 cloves garlic, crushed in a garlic press
1 celery stalk with leaves, diagonally sliced
1 small carrot, diagonally sliced
¹/₂ cup coarsely sliced fresh mushrooms
¹/₂ to 1 teaspoon dry mustard
¹/₂ cup small pineapple chunks
¹/₃ cup pineapple juice
2 teaspoons lime juice
¹/₄ cup low-sodium soy sauce
¹/₂ to 1 teaspoon grated fresh ginger
Salt and freshly ground pepper
1 to 3 sprigs fresh parsley, minced (optional)

Spray the bottom of a large, nonstick skillet with the cooking spray so that the ingredients will not stick to the skillet. Heat the skillet over medium-high heat. Evenly brown the pork for 5 minutes; stir frequently. Drain any excess fat.

Add the yellow and green onions, garlic, celery, carrot, and mushrooms; stir occasionally until the carrot is crisp-tender. Combine the mustard, pineapple, juices, soy sauce, and ginger in a small bowl; mix well. Stir the pineapple mixture into the skillet; heat for 2 minutes.

Place the warm, cooked pasta on oven-warmed plates. Serve the hot pork sauce over the pasta. Salt and pepper according to individual taste. Garnish the dish with the parsley.

4 servings

Each serving provides:

299	Calories	38 g	Carbohydrate
30 g	Protein	686 mg	Sodium
5 g	Fat	67 mg	Cholesterol

72

— ⚘ —

Chicken Monterey

Preparation time: 20 minutes
Cooking time: 16 to 25 minutes

This chicken dish served over wide ribbon noodles presents a light, downhome family-style chicken dinner. The simple, creamy cheese sauce coupled with a spicy anaheim chile creates a nutritious dish of real distinction and piquant flavor.

No stick cooking spray
1 ½ cups (about 3 ounces) dry wide ribbon noodles, cooked according to package directions, drained, and rinsed
³/₄ pound extra-lean chicken breasts, skinned and boned (about 4 small breast pieces)
1 small yellow onion, chopped
½ cup julienned green onions
1 to 2 cloves garlic, crushed in a garlic press
¼ to 1 small fresh anaheim or jalapeño chile, seeded, washed, and finely chopped (optional, for a spicier dish)
½ cup nonfat sour cream
1 cup low-sodium chicken broth
2 teaspoons flour
1 to 2 teaspoons minced fresh sage leaves
¼ cup grated lowfat Monterey Jack cheese
Salt and freshly ground pepper
1 to 3 sprigs fresh parsley or cilantro, minced (optional)

Spray the bottom of a large, nonstick skillet with the cooking spray so that the ingredients will not stick to the skillet. Heat the skillet over medium-high heat. Evenly brown the chicken breasts to lock in the juices; cook until golden brown, about 3 to 5 minutes per side. Reduce the heat to low. Cover; simmer the chicken in the skillet for 10 to 15 minutes. The chicken is done when it pulls apart with a fork.

Heat a nonstick medium saucepan over medium-high heat. Sauté the yellow and green onions, garlic, and chile until the onions are tender; stir frequently. Combine the sour cream, broth, flour, and sage in a bowl; mix well. Add the sour cream mixture to the saucepan; stir until the sauce thickens. Reduce the heat to low. Stir in the cheese; stir until the cheese melts. Salt and pepper the sauce according to individual taste.

Place the warm, cooked pasta on oven-warmed plates. Arrange a chicken breast on each plate of pasta. Evenly pour the creamy sauce over the pasta and chicken. Garnish the dish with the minced parsley or cilantro.

4 servings

Each serving provides:

282	Calories	25 g	Carbohydrate
34 g	Protein	208 mg	Sodium
5 g	Fat	82 mg	Cholesterol

73

—❀—

Beef Fricassee and Pasta

Preparation time: 30 minutes

The visual appeal of chunks of beef and pasta soaked in a rich, dark-brown sauce will immediately captivate and arouse your senses. The red wine is the heart of this recipe and subtly elicits the essence of a rich-flavored sauce. For extra appeal, serve this savory dish with a sprig of rosemary as garnish.

No stick cooking spray
4 ounces dry rigate, rigatoni, or mostaccioli pasta, cooked
    according to package directions, drained, and rinsed
³/₄ pound extra-lean round steak, cut across the grain into
    2-inch medallions (about 1 ¹/₂ cups)
1 small yellow onion, chopped
1 to 2 cloves garlic, crushed in a garlic press
1 celery stalk with leaves, sliced
1 bay leaf
1 small carrot, sliced
1 medium-size ripe tomato, finely chopped
1 cup fresh mushroom caps
¹/₃ cup red wine
2 teaspoons flour
1 ¹/₂ cups low-sodium beef broth
1 to 2 teaspoons minced fresh oregano leaves
Salt and freshly ground pepper

Spray the bottom of a 5-quart pot with the cooking spray so that the ingredients will not stick to the pot. Heat the pot over medium-high heat. Evenly brown the beef for 5 minutes; stir frequently. Drain any excess fat.

Add the onion, garlic, celery, bay leaf, carrot, tomato, and mushrooms. Cook until the carrot slices are crisp-tender; stir frequently. Combine the wine, flour, broth, and oregano in a small bowl; mix well. Stir the wine mixture into the pot; stir until the sauce thickens.

Bring the mixture to a boil. Reduce the heat to low. Simmer for 5 minutes; stir occasionally. Salt and pepper the dish according to individual taste. Remove the bay leaf. Stir in the cooked pasta just before serving; combine well. Serve the hot dish immediately.

4 servings

Each serving provides:

293	Calories	30 g	Carbohydrate
30 g	Protein	82 mg	Sodium
5 g	Fat	59 mg	Cholesterol

74

Pork in Spicy Tomato Sauce

Preparation time: 20 minutes
Cooking time: 10 to 15 minutes

When you taste the spiral-shaped pasta and chunks of pork saturated in a thick, wholesome tomato sauce, you will remember why you love pasta so much. If you are a chile con carne lover, you might like to try adding chile powder or sprigs of cilantro for a similar, spicy Mexican flavor.

No stick cooking spray
1 ½ cups (about 3 ounces) dry wide ribbon noodles or
    fettucine, cooked according to package directions,
    drained, and rinsed
³/₄ pound lean loin of pork, cut into 1 ½-inch cubes
    (about 1 ½ cups)
1 small yellow onion, sliced
1 to 2 cloves garlic, crushed in a garlic press
¼ to 1 small fresh anaheim chile, diced (optional, for
    spicier dish)
½ cup fresh corn kernels, uncooked (about 1 ear)
1 small ripe tomato, chopped
1 ½ cups tomato sauce
1 to 2 teaspoons minced fresh oregano leaves
1 to 2 teaspoons minced fresh marjoram leaves
Salt and freshly ground pepper

Spray the bottom of a 5-quart pot with the cooking spray so that the ingredients will not stick to the skillet. Heat the pot over medium-high heat. Evenly brown the pork to lock in the juices; stir frequently for 4 to 5 minutes. Drain any excess fat.

Add the onion, garlic, anaheim chile, corn, and tomato. Cook until the onions are tender; stir frequently. Stir in the tomato sauce, oregano, and marjoram; combine well. Reduce the heat to low. Simmer for 10 to 15 minutes; stir occasionally. Stir in the cooked pasta just before serving; combine well. Salt and pepper the dish according to individual taste. Serve the hot dish immediately.

4 servings

Each serving provides:

283	Calories	31 g	Carbohydrate
29 g	Protein	72 mg	Sodium
5 g	Fat	67 mg	Cholesterol

75

Chicken à la King

Preparation time: 25 minutes

Try the richness of a thick, creamy sauce with this easy-to-prepare chicken and vegetable combination. The snow peas are a great nutritional addition. They provide enough vitamin C to meet 100% of the daily nutritional requirement.

No stick cooking spray
2 cups (about 4 ounces) dry ziti pasta, cooked according to package directions, drained, and rinsed
$^3/_4$ pound extra-lean chicken, skinned, boned, and cut into tenderloin pieces (about 1 $^1/_2$ cups)
1 small yellow onion, chopped
$^1/_2$ cup finely minced green onions
1 to 2 cloves garlic, crushed in a garlic press
1 celery stalk with leaves, finely sliced
$^1/_2$ cup fresh snow peas
$^1/_2$ cup sliced fresh mushrooms
$^1/_2$ cup nonfat milk
2 teaspoons flour
$^1/_2$ cup nonfat sour cream
$^1/_2$ cup low-sodium chicken broth
1 to 2 sprigs fresh thyme, crushed without the stem
Salt and freshly ground pepper
1 to 3 sprigs fresh parsley, minced (optional)

Spray the bottom of a large, nonstick skillet with the cooking spray so that the ingredients will not stick to the skillet. Heat the skillet over medium-high heat. Evenly brown the chicken to lock in the juices; cook until golden brown, about 2 to 4 minutes per side.

Add the yellow and green onions, garlic, celery, peas, and mushrooms; stir frequently until the onions are tender. Combine the milk, flour, sour cream, broth, and thyme in a small bowl; mix well. Add the milk mixture to the skillet; stir constantly until the sauce thickens. Place the warm, cooked pasta on oven-warmed plates. Evenly spread the hot chicken sauce over the pasta. Salt and pepper according to individual taste. Garnish the dish with the parsley.

4 servings

Each serving provides:

269	Calories	54 g	Carbohydrate
38 g	Protein	132 mg	Sodium
3 g	Fat	72 mg	Cholesterol

76

—❦—

Chicken Alfredo

Preparation time: 20 minutes
Cooking time: 16 to 20 minutes

The addition of chicken makes this pasta dish extra nutritious, hearty, and flavorful. Try this classic Alfredo recipe if you want fewer calories and less fat than similar recipes. Other noodles that you might like to try with this recipe are mini-lasagne, rigatoni, or penne pasta. For a flavorful variation, try adding 2 tablespoons nonfat buttermilk (25 calories per ¼ cup) instead of 2 tablespoons sour cream to the sauce.

No stick cooking spray
4 ounces dry fettucine pasta, cooked according to package
    directions, drained, and rinsed
¾ pound extra-lean chicken, skinned, boned, and cut into
    tenderloin pieces (about 1 ½ cups)
1 small yellow onion, chopped
½ cup finely minced green onions
1 to 2 cloves garlic, crushed in a garlic press
1 ¼ cups nonfat sour cream
¼ cup grated nonfat Parmesan cheese
1 to 2 sprigs fresh thyme, crushed without the stems
Dash of fresh nutmeg
Salt and freshly ground pepper
1 to 3 sprigs fresh parsley or cilantro, minced (optional)

Spray the bottom of a large, nonstick skillet with the cooking spray so that the ingredients will not stick to the skillet. Heat the skillet over medium-high heat. Evenly brown the chicken to lock in the juices; cook until golden brown, about 3 to 5 minutes per side. Reduce the heat to low. Cover; simmer the chicken in the skillet for 10 minutes. The chicken is done when it pulls apart with a fork.

Heat a small saucepan over medium-high heat. Sauté the yellow and green onions and garlic until the onions are tender; stir frequently. Reduce the heat to low. Stir in the sour cream, Parmesan, thyme, and nutmeg; stir for 2 minutes. Salt and pepper the sauce according to individual taste.

Smother the chicken pieces in the sauce. Place the warm, cooked pasta on oven-warmed plates. Pour the hot chicken sauce over the pasta. Garnish the dish with the parsley or cilantro.

4 servings

Each serving provides:

294	Calories	60 g	Carbohydrate
43 g	Protein	72 mg	Sodium
3 g	Fat	237 mg	Cholesterol

77

---✇---

Herbed Flavored Chicken
over Spaghetti

Preparation time: 15 minutes
Cooking time: 16 to 25 minutes

Chicken and spaghetti lovers will go overboard for this
pasta dish topped with chicken coated in herbs and
Parmesan cheese. It is hard to believe something so good
can have so few calories. If you prefer, add lemon juice for
an extra tropical flavor or cayenne pepper for additional
spice. For a thicker, richer sauce, you might like to add
nonfat sour cream (30 calories per tablespoon).

No stick cooking spray
4 ounces dry thin spaghetti pasta, cooked according to
      package directions, drained, and rinsed
1 tablespoon flour
1/4 cup grated nonfat Parmesan cheese
1 to 3 sprigs fresh thyme, crushed without the stems
1 to 2 teaspoons minced fresh marjoram leaves
1 to 3 sprigs fresh parsley or cilantro, minced
1 pound extra-lean chicken breasts, skinned and boned
      (about 4 breast pieces)
1 small yellow onion, chopped
1/2 cup julienned green onions
1 to 2 cloves garlic, crushed in a garlic press
1 cup low-sodium chicken broth
1 cup water
Salt and freshly ground pepper

Place the flour, Parmesan cheese, thyme, marjoram, and parsley in a small paper bag. Clean the chicken in cold water; pat dry. Shake each chicken breast in the paper bag, one at a time, to coat each piece. Reserve the contents of the paper bag.

Spray the bottom of a large, nonstick skillet with the cooking spray so that the ingredients will not stick to the skillet. Heat the skillet over medium-high heat. Evenly brown the chicken breasts in the skillet to lock in the juices; cook until golden brown, about 3 to 5 minutes per side. Reduce the heat to low. Cover; simmer, turning the chicken once, for 10 to 15 minutes. The chicken is done when it pulls apart with a fork. Remove the chicken from the skillet.

In a medium-size saucepan over medium-high heat, sauté the yellow and green onions and garlic until the onions are tender; stir frequently. Add the broth, water, and reserved contents of the paper bag; stir 2 minutes until the ingredients are well combined. Salt and pepper the sauce according to individual taste. Place the warm, cooked pasta on oven-warmed plates. Arrange the chicken breasts on each plate of pasta. Pour the hot broth over the chicken and pasta.

4 servings

Each serving provides:			
291	Calories	60 g	Carbohydrate
48 g	Protein	96 mg	Sodium
4 g	Fat	145 mg	Cholesterol

78

※

Chicken Cacciatore

Preparation time: 25 minutes

This simple recipe, packed with superflavor, is an Italian classic and creates a wholesome, low-calorie family dinner. Nothing accents pasta quite like ripe tomatoes and fresh, green herbs. For a new twist to this recipe, try experimenting with different types of mushrooms, such as shiitake, enoki, or portabello.

No stick cooking spray
2 cups (about 4 ounces) dry mini-lasagne pasta, cooked according to package directions, drained, and rinsed
³/₄ pound extra-lean chicken, skinned, boned, and cut into large tenderloin pieces (about 1 ¹/₂ cups)
1 small yellow onion, finely sliced
¹/₂ cup finely minced green onions
1 to 2 cloves garlic, crushed in a garlic press
1 cup sliced fresh mushrooms
1 ¹/₂ cups tomato sauce
¹/₃ cup white wine
1 to 2 teaspoons minced fresh basil leaves
1 to 2 teaspoons minced fresh oregano leaves
1 bay leaf
Salt and freshly ground pepper
1 to 3 sprigs fresh parsley, minced (optional)

Spray the bottom of a large, nonstick skillet with the cooking spray so that the ingredients will not stick to the skillet. Heat the skillet over medium-high heat. Evenly brown the chicken to lock in the juices; cook until golden brown, about 2 to 4 minutes per side.

Add the yellow and green onions, garlic, and mushrooms; stir frequently until the onions are tender. Stir in the tomato sauce, wine, basil, oregano, and bay leaf; combine well. Reduce the heat to low. Cover; simmer for 2 minutes. Salt and pepper the sauce according to individual taste. The chicken is done when it pulls apart with a fork. Remove the bay leaf from the sauce.

Place the warm, cooked pasta on oven-warmed plates. Pour the hot chicken sauce over the pasta. Garnish the dish with the parsley.

4 servings

Each serving provides:

278	Calories	55 g	Carbohydrate
37 g	Protein	72 mg	Sodium
3 g	Fat	103 mg	Cholesterol

79

— ❧ —

Spicy Stripped Beef and Pineapple

Preparation time: 20 minutes

This beef dish has the sweet tangy flavor of pineapple blended with ginger and soy sauce. The strips of beef and vegetables combine to create a colorful, nutritious pasta dish served over the delicate lace of angel hair pasta. You can easily substitute other types of beef, poultry, or seafood for the beef used in this recipe.

No stick cooking spray
4 ounces dry angel hair pasta, cooked according to
       package directions, drained, and rinsed
½ pound extra-lean beef, cut into 1 ½-inch strips
       (about 1 cup)
1 small yellow onion, chopped
1 to 2 cloves garlic, crushed in a garlic press
8 to 9 fresh broccoli florets, cut into quarters
1 celery stalk, sliced
¼ to 1 small fresh anaheim chile, diced (optional, for
       spicier dish)
½ cup chopped pineapple
⅓ cup pineapple juice
¼ cup low-sodium soy sauce
¾ cup low-sodium beef broth
1 to 2 teaspoons grated fresh ginger
Salt and freshly ground pepper

Spray the bottom of a large, nonstick skillet with the cooking spray so that the ingredients will not stick to the skillet. Heat the skillet over medium-high heat. Evenly brown the beef for 5 minutes; stir frequently. Drain any excess fat.

Add the onion, garlic, broccoli, celery, and anaheim chile. Sauté until the broccoli is crisp-tender; stir occasionally. Stir in the pineapple, pineapple juice, soy sauce, broth, and ginger; combine well. Reduce the heat to low. Simmer for 2 minutes.

Stir in the warm cooked pasta just before serving; combine well. Salt and pepper the dish according to individual taste. Serve the hot pasta dish immediately.

4 servings

Each serving provides:

299	Calories	39 g	Carbohydrate
23 g	Protein	667 mg	Sodium
4 g	Fat	39 mg	Cholesterol

80

—✺—

Beef Stroganoff

Preparation time: 20 minutes

It's hard to believe that this fantastic dish is so easy to prepare and low in calories. A dash of sweet nutmeg or diced
green chile adds a new dimension to this light classical
dish served over warm ribbon noodles. Vegetarians can
create a veggie-version of this lowfat stroganoff recipe
using broccoli or other vegetables instead of the beef strips.

No stick cooking spray
2 cups (about 4 ounces) dry wide ribbon noodles, cooked
    according to package directions, drained, and rinsed
$^1/_2$ pound extra-lean beef, cut into 1 $^1/_2$-inch strips
    (about 1 cup)
1 small yellow onion, thinly sliced
$^1/_2$ cup finely minced green onions
1 to 2 cloves garlic, crushed in a garlic press
1 cup sliced mushrooms
1 $^1/_2$ cups nonfat sour cream
$^1/_2$ teaspoon Worcestershire sauce
$^1/_4$ to $^1/_2$ teaspoon nutmeg
Salt and freshly ground pepper
1 to 3 sprigs fresh parsley, minced (optional)

Spray the bottom of a large, nonstick skillet with the cooking spray so that the ingredients will not stick to the skillet. Heat the skillet over medium-high heat. Evenly brown the beef for 5 minutes; stir frequently. Drain any excess fat.

Add the yellow and green onions, garlic, and mushrooms. Sauté until the onions are tender; stir occasionally. Reduce the heat to low. Stir in the sour cream, Worcestershire, and nutmeg; combine well. Simmer for 2 minutes. Salt and pepper the dish according to individual taste.

Place the warm, cooked pasta on oven-warmed plates. Serve the beef and sour cream sauce over the pasta. Garnish the dish with the parsley.

4 servings

Each serving provides:

281	Calories	34 g	Carbohydrate
27 g	Protein	191 mg	Sodium
3 g	Fat	40 mg	Cholesterol

81

Beef Medallions over Wide Ribbon Noodles

Preparation time: 20 minutes

This hearty, easy-to-make beef recipe generously combines the flavors of meat, mushrooms, and tomatoes to
create a memorable dish of contrasting flavors, colors,
and textures. Lean lamb and pork are delicious alternative
choices instead of the round steak suggested in this recipe.
For a sensational variation, I like to add basil or oregano
leaves for even more enticing flavor.

No stick cooking spray
2 cups (about 4 ounces) dry ribbon noodles, cooked
    according to package directions, drained, and rinsed
³/₄ pound extra-lean round steak, trimmed, boned, and cut
    into 2-inch medallions (about 1 ½ cups)
1 small yellow onion, chopped
½ cup finely minced green onions
1 to 2 cloves garlic, crushed in a garlic press
1 cup sliced mushrooms
1 medium-size ripe tomato, finely chopped
Salt and freshly ground pepper
2 tablespoons grated nonfat Parmesan cheese

Spray the bottom of a large, nonstick skillet with the cooking spray so that the ingredients will not stick to the skillet. Heat the skillet over medium-high heat. Evenly brown the beef for 5 minutes; stir frequently. Drain any excess fat.

Stir in the yellow and green onions, garlic, mushrooms, and tomato; combine well. Sauté until the meat cooks thoroughly and the onions are tender; stir frequently. Salt and pepper the dish according to individual taste.

Place the warm, cooked pasta on oven-warmed plates. Serve the hot sauce over the pasta. Garnish the dish with the Parmesan cheese.

4 servings

Each serving provides:

278	Calories	28 g	Carbohydrate
31 g	Protein	82 mg	Sodium
5 g	Fat	59 mg	Cholesterol

82

—❦—

Grilled Chicken Strips

Preparation time: 15 minutes
Refrigeration time: 15 to 30 minutes
Grilling time: 6 to 10 minutes

Peaches impart a distinctive flavor to these chicken strips
served over a warm nest of pasta. For other recipe ideas,
you can substitute the peaches with pears, grapefruit,
apples, or grapes. If you cannot grill the chicken strips outdoors, you can also broil these pieces of chicken four to
five inches under the broiler or cook in a cast iron grill pan.

2 cups (about 4 ounces) dry penne pasta, cooked accord-
        ing to package directions, drained, and rinsed
2 tablespoons lime juice
1 tablespoon peach juice
1 tablespoon low-sodium soy sauce
2 teaspoons apple cider vinegar
1 pound extra-lean chicken breast halves, skinned, and
        boned (about 4 breast pieces)
$^1/_2$ small yellow onion, sliced
$^1/_2$ cup finely sliced green onions
1 to 2 cloves garlic, crushed in a garlic press
$^1/_2$ small red bell pepper, finely sliced
1 small ripe peach, finely chopped
1 cup low-sodium chicken broth
Salt and freshly ground pepper

Combine the lime and peach juices, soy sauce, and vinegar in a glass baking dish. Rub the chicken in the marinade to thoroughly coat the chicken with the juices. Cover; refrigerate the chicken breasts for 15 to 30 minutes; turn occasionally. Remove the chicken from the marinade; reserve the marinade.

Grill the chicken breasts four to five inches above a bed of hot coals for 3 to 5 minutes on each side. Grill until the chicken cooks thoroughly and the juices run clear. Cut each chicken breast into large strips.

Heat a medium-size saucepan over medium-high heat. Sauté the yellow and green onions, garlic, and red bell pepper until the onions are tender; stir frequently. Add the peach, broth, and reserved marinade to the saucepan. Bring the mixture to a boil; reduce the heat to low. Stir the cooked pasta into the saucepan just before serving; combine well. Salt and pepper the dish according to individual taste. Place the pasta on oven-warmed plates. Arrange the chicken strips on each plate of peaches and pasta.

4 servings

Each serving provides:

289	Calories	60 g	Carbohydrate
46 g	Protein	243 mg	Sodium
3 g	Fat	96 mg	Cholesterol

83

—❦—

Oriental Grilled Kabobs

Preparation time: 20 minutes
Refrigeration time: 15 to 30 minutes
Grilling time: 8 to 10 minutes

These kabobs have an oriental twist stemming from the
fused flavors of pineapple, soy sauce, and ginger. For a
delicious variation, substitute tofu or shrimp for the beef
suggested in this recipe. If you cannot grill outdoors, you
can also broil these pieces of beef four to five inches under
the broiler or cook in a cast iron grill pan.

5 ounces dry angel hair pasta, cooked according to
    package directions, drained, and rinsed
2 teaspoons apple cider vinegar
1 tablespoon low-sodium soy sauce
1 tablespoon lime juice
$1/4$ cup low-sodium beef broth
1 to 2 teaspoons grated fresh ginger
$1/2$ pound extra-lean beef, cut into large chunks
    (about 1 cup)
1 small zucchini, sliced into 1-inch chunks
4 cherry tomatoes, cut in half
8 small mushroom caps
8 pineapple chunks
$1/2$ small red bell pepper, sliced
$1/2$ cup julienned green onions

1 to 2 cloves garlic, crushed in a garlic press
1 teaspoon extra-virgin olive oil
Salt and freshly ground pepper

Combine the vinegar, soy sauce, lime juice, broth, and ginger in a glass baking dish. Toss the beef, zucchini, tomatoes, mushrooms, pineapple, and bell pepper in the marinade to thoroughly coat with the juices. Cover; marinate in the refrigerator for 15 to 30 minutes; turn the beef pieces occasionally.

Remove the beef from the marinade; reserve the marinade. Alternately skewer the beef, zucchini, tomatoes, mushrooms, pineapples, and bell pepper on the metal skewers. Grill the kabobs four to five inches above a bed of hot coals for 4 to 5 minutes on each side.

Heat a medium-size saucepan over medium-low heat. Sauté the reserved marinade, green onions, garlic, and oil for 1 minute. Reduce the heat to low. Stir the cooked pasta into the marinade just before serving; combine well. Salt and pepper the dish according to individual taste. Place the pasta on oven-warmed plates. Lay the grilled kabobs on top of the pasta.

4 servings

Each serving provides:

281	Calories	38 g	Carbohydrate
23 g	Protein	200 mg	Sodium
6 g	Fat	39 mg	Cholesterol

84

Pork and Cilantro over Rigatoni

Preparation time: 25 minutes

Cooks will love this delectable combination of pork, tomatoes, and cilantro. The chunks of pork, heavily soaked in a
spicy sauce, will satisfy your desire for the blended flavors
of chiles and pork. Quick and easy to prepare, this colorful, tempting pasta dish is particularly memorable when
eaten with a chunk of bread and a tossed green salad. If
you prefer, you can substitute other herbs, like rosemary
or parsley for the cilantro.

No stick cooking spray
1 ½ cups (about 3 ounces) dry rigatoni pasta, cooked ac-
    cording to package directions, drained, and rinsed
1 pound pork loin, trimmed, and diagonally sliced into
    thin strips (about 2 cups)
1 small yellow onion, quartered and cut into strips
½ cup julienned green onions
1 to 2 cloves garlic, crushed in a garlic press
¼ to 1 small fresh anaheim chile, seeded, washed, and
    finely chopped
½ small red bell pepper, cut into julienne strips
½ cup pineapple chunks
½ cup tomato sauce
¼ cup low-sodium beef broth
1 to 2 teaspoons minced fresh oregano leaves
Salt and freshly ground pepper
1 to 3 sprigs cilantro, minced

Spray the bottom of a large, nonstick skillet with the cooking spray so that the ingredients will not stick to the skillet. Heat the skillet over medium-high heat. Evenly brown the pork for 5 minutes; stir frequently. Drain any excess fat.

Add the yellow and green onions, garlic, anaheim chile, bell pepper, and pineapple. Stir frequently until the pork cooks thoroughly and the bell pepper is crisp-tender. Stir in the tomato sauce, broth, and oregano; combine well. Reduce the heat to low. Simmer for 2 to 4 minutes. Salt and pepper the dish according to individual taste.

Place the warm, cooked pasta on oven-warmed plates. Serve the hot pork sauce over the pasta. Garnish the dish with the cilantro.

4 servings

Each serving provides:

306	Calories	28 g	Carbohydrate
36 g	Protein	78 mg	Sodium
6 g	Fat	89 mg	Cholesterol

85

Tropical Pineapple Chicken

Preparation time: 20 minutes

You will love this irresistible, succulent delight featuring tangy-sweet fruit flavors. For additional island flair, you can add assorted fruits like seedless red grapes, strawberries, kiwis, or cherries. For a complete satisfying meal, serve this exotic tropical dish with a garden fresh salad.

No stick cooking spray
2 cups (about 4 ounces) dry wide egg noodles, cooked
    according to package directions, drained, and rinsed
³/₄ pound extra-lean chicken, skinned, boned, and cut into
    tenderloin pieces (about 1 ¹/₂ cups)
1 small yellow onion, chopped
¹/₂ cup finely sliced green onions
1 to 2 cloves garlic, crushed in a garlic press
¹/₂ small green bell pepper, sliced
¹/₂ medium-size banana, sliced
¹/₂ cup low-sodium chicken broth
³/₄ cup chopped pineapple (1 ¹/₂-inch pieces)
¹/₂ cup pineapple juice
1 teaspoon lime juice
Salt and freshly ground pepper

Spray the bottom of a large, nonstick skillet with the cooking spray so that the ingredients will not stick to the skillet. Heat the skillet over medium-high heat. Evenly brown the chicken to lock in the juices; cook until golden brown, about 2 to 4 minutes per side.

Add the yellow and green onions, garlic, and bell pepper. Sauté until the bell pepper is crisp-tender; stir frequently. Stir in the banana, broth, pineapple, and juices; combine well. Reduce the heat to low.

Stir in the cooked pasta just before serving; combine well. Salt and pepper the dish according to individual taste. Serve the hot chicken dish immediately.

4 servings

Each serving provides:			
285	Calories	68 g	Carbohydrate
36 g	Protein	74 mg	Sodium
3 g	Fat	72 mg	Cholesterol

86

—❧—

Indonesian Beef and Angel Hair Pasta

Preparation time: 25 minutes

Served with a heap of chewy, warm pasta, this dish is a quick-to-make combination of vegetables and beef that is full of contrasting flavors and colors. The Dijon-style flavoring adds an especially zippy twist. Enjoy this dish with a tossed green salad and fruit for dessert.

No stick cooking spray
4 ounces dry angel hair pasta, cooked according to
    package directions, drained, and rinsed
³/₄ pound round steak, trimmed, and diagonally sliced into
    thin strips (about 1 ¹/₂ cups)
1 small yellow onion, quartered and thickly sliced
¹/₂ cup julienned green onions
1 to 2 cloves garlic, crushed in a garlic press
¹/₂ small carrot, cut into julienne strips
¹/₂ small red bell pepper, cut into julienne strips
¹/₄ to 1 small fresh anaheim chile, seeded, washed, and
    finely chopped
¹/₃ cup low-sodium soy sauce
¹/₄ cup water

2 teaspoons peanut or sesame oil
1 to 2 teaspoons Dijon-style mustard
Salt and freshly ground pepper
Dash of cayenne pepper (optional, for a spicier dish)

Spray the bottom of a large, nonstick skillet with the cooking spray so that the ingredients will not stick to the skillet. Heat the skillet over medium-high heat. Evenly brown the beef for 5 minutes; stir frequently. Drain any excess fat.

Add the yellow and green onions, garlic, carrot, bell pepper, and anaheim chile. Sauté until the carrot strips are crisp-tender; stir frequently. Add the soy sauce, water, oil, and mustard; mix well. Stir in the cooked pasta just before serving; combine well. Salt and pepper the dish according to individual taste. Garnish the dish with the cayenne pepper. Serve the hot dish immediately.

4 servings

Each serving provides:

299	Calories	29 g	Carbohydrate
31 g	Protein	998 mg	Sodium
6 g	Fat	59 mg	Cholesterol

87

---❦---

Singapore Chicken over Vermicelli

Preparation time: 20 minutes

If you love the taste of sweet and sour, you will enjoy this blend of chicken, pineapple, and lime juice served over a delicate nest of pasta. The oriental and tropical flavoring turns this chicken favorite into an exotic treat! The carrots provide lots of vitamin A, brilliant color, and extra flavor.

No stick cooking spray
2 cups (about 4 ounces) dry vermicelli pasta, cooked
    according to package directions, drained, and rinsed
³/₄ pound extra-lean chicken, skinned, boned, and cut into
    tenderloin pieces (about 1 ¹/₂ cups)
1 small yellow onion, chopped
¹/₂ cup finely minced green onions
1 to 2 cloves garlic, crushed in a garlic press
1 celery stalk, diagonally sliced
¹/₂ small carrot, diagonally sliced
¹/₄ cup sliced water chestnuts
¹/₂ small red bell pepper, coarsely chopped
¹/₂ cup pineapple chunks
¹/₃ cup pineapple juice
2 teaspoons lime juice
¹/₃ cup low-sodium soy sauce

Dash of ginger
Salt and freshly ground pepper
1 to 3 sprigs fresh parsley, minced (optional)

Spray the bottom of a large, nonstick skillet with the cooking spray so that the ingredients will not stick to the skillet. Heat the skillet over medium-high heat. Evenly brown the chicken to lock in the juices; cook until golden brown, about 2 to 4 minutes per side stir. Reduce the heat to low.

Add the yellow and green onions, garlic, celery, carrot, water chestnuts, and bell pepper. Sauté until the carrot slices are crisp-tender; stir frequently. Stir in the pineapple, juices, soy sauce, and ginger; combine well. Salt and pepper the dish according to individual taste. Reduce the heat to low. Simmer for 2 minutes.

Place the warm, cooked pasta on oven-warmed plates. Serve the chicken sauce over the pasta. Garnish the dish with the parsley.

4 servings

Each serving provides:

297	Calories	44 g	Carbohydrate
31 g	Protein	992 mg	Sodium
3 g	Fat	72 mg	Cholesterol

88

─── ✿ ───

Spanish Chicken and Pasta

Preparation time: 10 minutes
Cooking time: 20 to 25 minutes

This is a pasta variation of a traditional Spanish chicken
and rice dish. It has an intriguing Spanish flair with brilliant colors and contrasting flavors. If you like spicy, you
will want to try this dish made with chiles and pasta
soaked in tomato sauce. Don't forget to add more chiles
if you like a spicier dish.

No stick cooking spray
1 ¼ pounds extra-lean chicken breasts, skinned and boned
    (about 4 breast pieces)
1 small yellow onion, chopped
½ cup finely sliced green onions
1 to 2 cloves garlic, crushed in a garlic press
½ cup chopped red bell pepper
¼ to 1 small fresh anaheim chile, seeded, washed, and
    finely chopped
1 medium-size ripe tomato, finely chopped
1 cup (2 ounces) dry fideo pasta, uncooked
1 cup tomato sauce
½ teaspoon lime juice
1 ½ cups low-sodium chicken broth
1 cup water
1 bay leaf

1 to 2 teaspoons minced fresh oregano leaves
Salt and freshly ground pepper
1 to 3 sprigs fresh parsley or cilantro, minced (optional)

Spray the bottom of a large, nonstick skillet with the cooking spray so that the ingredients will not stick to the skillet. Heat the skillet over medium-high heat. Evenly brown the chicken breasts to lock in the juices; cook until golden brown, about 3 to 5 minutes per side. Remove the chicken breasts.

Add the yellow and green onions, garlic, bell pepper, anaheim chile, tomato, and pasta to the skillet; stir frequently until the bell pepper softens. Stir in the tomato sauce, lime juice, broth, water, bay leaf, and oregano; combine well. Place the chicken breasts in the sauce. Reduce the heat to low.

Cover; simmer the chicken mixture for 20 to 25 minutes. The chicken is done when it cooks throughout and pulls apart with a fork. Add additional broth if the sauce cooks away. Remove the bay leaf. Salt and pepper the dish according to individual taste. Garnish the dish with the parsley or cilantro. Serve the hot dish immediately.

4 servings

Each serving provides:

282	Calories	57 g	Carbohydrate
51 g	Protein	114 mg	Sodium
5 g	Fat	108 mg	Cholesterol

Hot Baked Pasta Dishes in Minutes

89

—❦—

Stuffed Pasta Shells

Preparation time: 20 minutes
Baking time: 20 minutes
Preheat oven to 350°

Cooks will love this delectable casserole using a variation of pesto made with sour cream and mushrooms for stuffing. A rich, savory tomato sauce covers the pesto-stuffed shells and presents a colorful combination for everyone's enjoyment. If you want more color, use black olives as an especially attractive garnish. Ricotta cheese is a flavorful substitute in place of the sour cream.

No stick cooking spray
2 cups dry large seashell pasta, cooked according
    to package directions, drained, and rinsed
    (about 24 shells)
1 ¼ cups tomato sauce
1 to 2 cloves garlic, crushed in a garlic press
½ small yellow onion, chopped
½ cup chopped fresh mushrooms
1 cup nonfat sour cream
¼ cup grated nonfat Parmesan cheese
¼ to ½ cup minced fresh basil leaves
2 to 6 sprigs fresh parsley, minced
4 tablespoons grated lowfat mozzarella cheese
½ cup finely minced green onions
Salt and freshly ground pepper

Combine ¼ cup tomato sauce and the garlic, yellow onion, mushrooms, sour cream, Parmesan, basil, and parsley in a bowl; mix well. Stuff each cooked seashell with about 1 tablespoon of the filling.

Spray a glass, bake-proof baking dish with the cooking spray so that the ingredients will not stick to the dish. Place the stuffed shells in the baking dish. Pour the remaining 1 cup tomato sauce over the stuffed shells. Sprinkle the mozzarella cheese over the stuffed shells. Garnish the dish with the green onions. Salt and pepper the dish according to individual taste. Bake the dish in a preheated oven at 350° for 20 minutes. Serve the hot dish immediately.

4 servings

Each serving provides:

242	Calories	41 g	Carbohydrate
15 g	Protein	244 mg	Sodium
4 g	Fat	8 mg	Cholesterol

90

—❦—

Chicken and Mushroom Casserole

Preparation time: 20 minutes
Baking time: 15 minutes
Preheat oven to 350°

Got a busy schedule? Need to serve dinner fast? This is a
perfect make-ahead dish for the busy cook. For an enticing variation, substitute the Monterey Jack cheese with
grated lowfat mozzarella or Swiss cheese as the topping.

No stick cooking spray
2 cups (about 4 ounces) dry ribbon noodles, cooked
     according to package directions, drained, and rinsed
³/4 pound extra-lean chicken, skinned, boned, and cut into
     tenderloin pieces (about 1 ¹/2 cups)
1 small yellow onion, sliced into rings
1 to 2 cloves garlic, crushed in a garlic press
5 to 6 broccoli florets, cut in half
1 cup finely sliced fresh mushrooms
¹/4 cup nonfat sour cream
1 tablespoon flour
1 cup nonfat milk
2 to 4 sprigs fresh thyme, crushed without the stems
2 tablespoons grated lowfat Monterey Jack cheese
¹/4 cup finely minced green onions
Salt and freshly ground pepper

Spray the bottom of a large, nonstick skillet and glass baking dish with the cooking spray so that the ingredients will not stick to the skillet.

Heat the skillet over medium-high heat. In the skillet, evenly brown the chicken to lock in the juices; cook until golden brown, about 2 to 4 minutes per side. Add the onion, garlic, broccoli, and mushrooms. Sauté until the broccoli is crisp-tender; stir frequently.

Combine the sour cream, flour, milk, and thyme in a small bowl; mix well. Stir the milk mixture into the skillet; stir constantly until the sauce thickens.

Place the cooked pasta in the baking dish. Pour the chicken sauce over the pasta. Sprinkle the cheese and green onions over the casserole. Salt and pepper the dish according to individual taste. Heat the casserole in a preheated oven at 350° for 15 minutes. Serve the hot dish immediately.

4 servings

Each serving provides:

299	Calories	55 g	Carbohydrate
41 g	Protein	175 mg	Sodium
4 g	Fat	78 mg	Cholesterol

91

——❦——

Beef Lasagne Pie

Preparation time: 20 minutes
Baking time: 15 minutes
Preheat oven to 350°

Reshape an Italian tradition into a new light classic tradition. This is the perfect dish for an elegant meal or a more informal family dinner. For a healthy, light lunch, serve wedges of this special lasagne with family and friends. Complete your lasagne feast with a garden salad and a chunk of fresh bread.

No stick cooking spray
1 cup (about 2 ounces) dry mini-lasagne pasta, cooked
    according to package directions, drained, and rinsed
½ pound extra-lean ground round beef (about 1 cup)
1 small yellow onion, finely chopped
½ cup finely sliced green onions
1 to 2 cloves garlic, crushed in a garlic press
1 cup finely sliced fresh mushrooms
1 to 2 teaspoons minced fresh oregano leaves
2 to 3 sprigs fresh thyme, crushed without the stems
1 to 2 teaspoons minced fresh basil leaves
2 cups tomato sauce
¼ cup nonfat ricotta cheese
½ cup nonfat cottage cheese
¼ cup grated lowfat mozzarella cheese
Salt and freshly ground pepper

Spray the bottom of a large, nonstick skillet and a medium-size pie pan with the cooking spray so that the ingredients will not stick to the skillet.

Heat the skillet over medium-high heat. In the skillet, evenly brown the beef for 5 minutes; stir frequently. Drain any excess fat. Add the yellow and green onions, garlic, mushrooms, oregano, thyme, and basil. Sauté until the onions are tender; stir frequently. Stir in the tomato sauce; combine well.

Place the cooked pasta in the pie pan. Spread the ricotta and cottage cheese on the pasta. Pour the tomato sauce over the top. Sprinkle the mozzarella cheese over the casserole. Salt and pepper the dish according to individual taste. Bake the lasagne pie uncovered in a preheated oven at 350° for 15 minutes. Serve the hot dish immediately.

5 servings

Each serving provides:

286	Calories	29 g	Carbohydrate
20 g	Protein	307 mg	Sodium
11 g	Fat	38 mg	Cholesterol

92

——✣——

Breasts of Chicken in Tomato Sauce

Preparation time: 20 minutes
Cooking time: 15 to 20 minutes

Chicken and Italian-style tomato sauce combine to set this savory, easy-to-make casserole apart from the ordinary fare. The tomato sauce adds the perfect touch of exotic, piquant flavor to your favorite pasta. This dish goes well with a vegetable side dish or a garden fresh salad. For richer flavor, you might like to try adding red wine (about 25 calories per fluid ounce).

No stick cooking spray
4 extra-lean chicken breasts, skinned and boned
    (about 1 pound)
1 small yellow onion, sliced into rings
1/2 cup finely minced green onions
1 to 2 cloves garlic, crushed in a garlic press
1/2 cup fresh mushroom caps, stems removed
1 cup tomato sauce
1 1/2 cups low-sodium chicken broth
1 to 2 teaspoons minced fresh oregano leaves
1 to 2 teaspoons minced fresh basil leaves
2 cups (about 4 ounces) dry ribbon noodles, uncooked
Salt and freshly ground pepper

Spray the bottom of a large, covered, flameproof casserole with the cooking spray so that the ingredients will not stick to the casserole. Heat the casserole over medium-high heat. Evenly brown the chicken to lock in the juices; cook until golden brown, about 2 to 4 minutes per side. Remove the chicken breasts.

Stir in the yellow and green onions, garlic, and mushrooms. Sauté until the onions are tender; stir frequently. Stir in the tomato sauce, broth, oregano, and basil; combine well. Smother the pasta in the casserole with the sauce. Place the chicken on top of the pasta and sauce. Reduce the heat to low.

Cover; simmer the chicken mixture for 15 to 20 minutes. The chicken is done when it pulls apart with a fork. Salt and pepper the chicken dish according to individual taste. Serve the hot dish immediately.

4 servings

Each serving provides:

297	Calories	29 g	Carbohydrate
37 g	Protein	100 mg	Sodium
4 g	Fat	96 mg	Cholesterol

93

— ❦ —

Vegetable and Beef Casserole

Preparation time: 20 minutes
Baking time: 15 minutes
Preheat oven to 350°

Vegetables and beef combine to make the perfect casserole.
Make this dish in advance, grab it from the freezer, and
warm it in the oven while you relax before dinner. This
casserole has pasta, vegetables, and beef in a one-dish meal
that is fast, easy to prepare, and wonderful to eat.

No stick cooking spray
1 ½ cups (about 3 ounces) dry rotelle pasta, cooked
     according to package directions, drained, and rinsed
½ pound extra-lean ground round beef (about 1 cup)
1 small yellow onion, finely chopped
1 to 2 cloves garlic, crushed in a garlic press
1 celery stalk with leaves, finely sliced
½ cup corn kernels
9 to 12 fresh cauliflower florets, cut in half
2 cups tomato sauce
1 to 2 teaspoons minced fresh marjoram leaves
1 to 2 teaspoons minced fresh basil leaves
3 tablespoons grated lowfat Monterey Jack cheese
Salt and freshly ground pepper

Spray the bottom of a large, nonstick skillet and medium-size casserole with the cooking spray so that the ingredients will not stick to the skillet.

Heat the skillet over medium-high heat. Evenly brown the beef for 5 minutes; stir frequently. Drain any excess fat. Add the onion, garlic, celery, corn, and cauliflower. Sauté the vegetables until the cauliflower is crisp-tender; stir frequently. Stir in the tomato sauce, marjoram, and basil; combine well.

Place the cooked pasta in the casserole. Spread the beef and tomato sauce over the pasta. Sprinkle the cheese over the casserole. Salt and pepper the dish according to individual taste. Bake the casserole uncovered in a preheated oven at 350° for 15 minutes. Serve the hot dish immediately.

4 servings

Each serving provides:

278	Calories	37 g	Carbohydrate
21 g	Protein	175 mg	Sodium
14 g	Fat	48 mg	Cholesterol

94

— ❦ —

Eggplant Parmeſan Caſſerole

Preparation time: 15 minuteſ
Baking time: 15 minuteſ
Preheat oven to 350°

Taken piping hot from the oven, this simmering casserole
offers mouth-watering appeal. A topping of Parmesan
cheese adds the final kick of flavor. For a healthy, light
lunch, serve smaller portions of this casserole with a slice
of toast.

No stick cooking spray
2 cups (about 4 ounces) dry ribbon noodles, cooked ac-
    cording to package directions, drained, and rinsed
1 teaspoon extra-virgin olive oil
1 small yellow onion, finely chopped
½ cup finely sliced green onions
1 to 2 cloves garlic, crushed in a garlic press
1 cup sliced eggplant
1 cup finely sliced fresh mushrooms
2 cups tomato sauce
1 to 2 teaspoons minced fresh oregano leaves
1 to 2 teaspoons minced fresh basil leaves
¼ cup nonfat cottage cheese
¼ cup nonfat ricotta cheese
2 tablespoons grated nonfat Parmesan cheese
3 tablespoons grated lowfat mozzarella cheese
Salt and freshly ground pepper

Heat the oil in a large, nonstick skillet over medium-high heat. Sauté the yellow and green onions, garlic, eggplant, and mushrooms until the eggplant is tender; stir frequently. Stir in the tomato sauce, oregano, and basil; mix well. Reduce the heat to low.

Spray a casserole with the cooking spray so that the ingredients will not stick to the bottom. Place the cooked pasta in the casserole. Evenly spread the cottage and ricotta cheeses over the pasta. Pour the sauce over the dish. Sprinkle the Parmesan and mozzarella cheeses over the casserole. Salt and pepper the dish according to individual taste. Bake the casserole uncovered in a preheated oven at 350° for 15 minutes. Serve the hot dish immediately.

4 servings

	Each serving provides:		
191	Calories	36 g	Carbohydrate
10 g	Protein	159 mg	Sodium
2 g	Fat	1 mg	Cholesterol

95

Stuffed Manicotti

Preparation time: 20 minutes
Baking time: 20 minutes
Preheat oven to 350°

Stuffed manicotti is an attractive, deliciously different, and healthful way to capture the savory appeal of a rich tomato sauce. The pasta shells gain hearty, rich flavor from a stuffing of different cheeses. Try other sauces or herbs with these stuffed shells.

No stick cooking spray
4 manicotti shells, cooked according to package
    directions, drained, and rinsed
1 ¼ cups tomato sauce
1 to 2 cloves garlic, crushed in a garlic press
1 cup sliced fresh mushrooms
1 tablespoon grated nonfat Parmesan cheese
½ cup nonfat cottage cheese
¼ cup nonfat ricotta cheese
1 to 2 teaspoons minced fresh oregano leaves
2 to 3 sprigs fresh thyme, crushed without the stems
4 tablespoons grated lowfat mozzarella cheese
¼ cup chopped black olives
½ cup finely minced green onions
Salt and freshly ground pepper

Combine ¼ cup of the tomato sauce and the garlic, mush-rooms, Parmesan, cottage and ricotta cheeses, oregano, and thyme in a bowl. Reserve ⅕ of the filling. Stuff the cooked pasta shells with the remaining filling.

Spray a glass, bake-proof baking dish with the cooking spray so that the ingredients will not stick to the bottom. Place the stuffed shells in the baking dish. Spread the remaining 1 cup tomato sauce over the stuffed shells. Evenly spread the reserved filling over the stuffed shells. Sprinkle the mozzarella cheese over the casserole. Garnish the dish with the black olives and green onions. Bake the dish in a preheated oven at 350° for 20 minutes. Salt and pepper according to individual taste. Serve the hot dish immediately.

4 servings

Each serving provides:

238	Calories	32 g	Carbohydrate
15 g	Protein	416 mg	Sodium
6 g	Fat	13 mg	Cholesterol

96

—❦—

Tuna Spring Casserole

Preparation time: 20 minutes
Baking time: 15 minutes
Preheat oven to 350°

Nutritious foods can make the difference. This perfectly seasoned casserole will stimulate and satisfy the appetite with nourishing and flavorful ingredients. For an attractive variation, use dried bread crumbs or chopped olives as a special topping. A tuna casserole is the perfect recipe for an appetizing buffet, special meal for friends, or a quick meal made in minutes.

No stick cooking spray
2 cups (about 4 ounces) dry rotini pasta, cooked
    according to package directions, drained, and rinsed
1 small yellow onion, finely sliced into rings
½ cup finely sliced green onions
1 to 2 cloves garlic, crushed in a garlic press
1 celery stalk with leaves, finely sliced
½ cup corn kernels
½ cup finely sliced fresh mushrooms
½ pound fresh tuna, coarsely cut into 1½-inch chunks
    (about 1 cup)
½ cup nonfat sour cream
½ cup nonfat milk
2 teaspoons flour
½ cup low-sodium vegetable or fish broth

2 to 3 sprigs fresh thyme, crushed without the stems
1 to 2 teaspoons minced fresh marjoram leaves
3 tablespoons grated lowfat Monterey Jack cheese
Salt and freshly ground pepper

Spray the bottom of a large, nonstick skillet and medium-size casserole with the cooking spray so that the ingredients will not stick to the skillet. Heat the skillet over medium-high heat. In the skillet, sauté the yellow and green onions, garlic, celery, corn, mushrooms, and tuna until the celery is crisp-tender; stir frequently.

Combine the sour cream, milk, flour, broth, thyme, and marjoram in a small bowl; mix well. Stir the sour cream mixture into the skillet; stir constantly until the sauce thickens.

Place the cooked pasta in the casserole. Spread the tuna mixture over the pasta. Sprinkle the cheese over the casserole. Salt and pepper the dish according to individual taste. Bake the casserole uncovered in a preheated oven at 350° for 15 minutes. Serve the hot dish immediately.

4 servings

Each serving provides:

276	Calories	34 g	Carbohydrate
25 g	Protein	175 mg	Sodium
3 g	Fat	34 mg	Cholesterol

97

—✥—

Broccoli, Mushroom, and Ham Casserole

Preparation time: 20 minutes
Baking time: 15 minutes
Preheat oven to 350°

This recipe combines broccoli, mushrooms, and ham in a simple cream sauce for a one-dish meal that is fast, delicious, and easy to prepare. The contrast of broccoli and ham adds great taste appeal. In this low-calorie casserole, the milk keeps the ham moist and the vegetables succulent.

No stick cooking spray
2 cups (about 4 ounces) dry rigate pasta, cooked
     according to package directions, drained, and rinsed
1 small yellow onion, finely chopped
$^1/_2$ cup finely sliced green onions
1 to 2 cloves garlic, crushed in a garlic press
7 to 8 broccoli florets, cut in half
$^1/_2$ small red bell pepper, cut into julienne strips
1 cup finely sliced mushrooms
1 cup coarsely chopped, cooked ham
1 cup nonfat milk
4 teaspoons flour
1 to 2 teaspoons minced fresh marjoram leaves

2 to 3 sprigs fresh thyme, crushed without the stems
3 tablespoons grated lowfat Monterey Jack cheese
Salt and freshly ground pepper

Heat a large, nonstick skillet over medium-high heat.
Sauté the yellow and green onions, garlic, broccoli, bell
pepper, mushrooms, and ham until the broccoli is crisp-
tender; stir frequently. Combine the milk, flour, marjoram,
and thyme in a small bowl; mix well. Add the milk mixture
to the skillet; stir constantly until the sauce thickens.
    Spray a casserole with the cooking spray so that the
ingredients will not stick to the bottom. Place the cooked
pasta in the casserole. Spread the ham mixture over the
pasta. Sprinkle the cheese over the casserole. Salt and
pepper according to individual taste. Bake the casserole
uncovered in a preheated oven at 350° for 15 minutes.
Serve the hot dish immediately.

4 servings

Each serving provides:

285	Calories	31 g	Carbohydrate
23 g	Protein	141 mg	Sodium
0 g	Fat	50 mg	Cholesterol

98

—✥—

Mini-Lasagne Vegetable Casserole

Preparation time: 20 minutes
Baking time: 20 minutes
Preheat oven to 350°

Everyone loves lasagne! Here is a light version of a classic Italian recipe for lasagne lovers. This special vegetable lasagne dish is big on flavor and nutritional ingredients and low on calories and fat. Serve smaller portions for lunch with a chunk of Italian bread.

No stick cooking spray
2 cups (about 4 ounces) dry mini-lasagne pasta, cooked
    according to package directions, drained, and rinsed
1 small yellow onion, finely chopped
1/2 cup finely sliced green onions
1 to 2 cloves garlic, crushed in a garlic press
1/2 small zucchini, sliced
6 to 7 small cauliflower florets
1/2 cup finely sliced mushrooms
2 cups tomato sauce
1 to 2 teaspoons minced fresh oregano leaves
1 to 2 teaspoons minced fresh marjoram leaves
1/4 cup nonfat cottage cheese
1/4 cup nonfat ricotta cheese
1/4 cup grated lowfat mozzarella cheese
Salt and freshly ground pepper

Heat a large, nonstick skillet over medium-high heat. Sauté the yellow and green onions, garlic, zucchini, cauliflower, and mushrooms until the cauliflower is crisp-tender; stir frequently. Stir in the tomato sauce, oregano, and marjoram; reduce the heat to low. Simmer the sauce for 3 to 5 minutes; stir occasionally.

Spray the bottom of a glass baking dish with the cooking spray so that the ingredients will not stick to the bottom. Place the cooked pasta in the baking dish. Spread the cottage and ricotta cheeses over the pasta. Pour the sauce over the top. Sprinkle the mozzarella cheese over the casserole. Salt and pepper the dish according to individual taste. Bake the casserole uncovered in a pre-heated oven at 350° for 20 minutes. Serve the hot dish immediately.

4 servings

Each serving provides:

218	Calories	35 g	Carbohydrate
14 g	Protein	190 mg	Sodium
3 g	Fat	10 mg	Cholesterol

99

_⸎_

Seafood Tetrazzini

Preparation time: 15 minutes
Baking time: 15 minutes
Preheat oven to 350°

Seafood lovers will enjoy the smooth blend of a creamy, flavorful white sauce with an appetizing assortment of seafood. Served over rigatoni noodles, this casserole will get your attention and give your taste buds instant satisfaction. Wine lovers might like to add a few tablespoons of dry white wine for additional flavor.

No stick cooking spray
2 cups (about 4 ounces) dry rigatoni or rigate pasta,
    cooked according to package directions, drained, and
    rinsed
1 small yellow onion, finely chopped
½ cup finely sliced green onions
1 to 2 cloves garlic, crushed in a garlic press
¼ pound fresh firm, white fish, cut into small chunks
    (about ½ cup)
¼ pound fresh large shrimp, peeled, deveined, and
    cleaned (about ½ cup)
¼ pound fresh small scallops, mussels, or clams, cleaned
    in cold water (about ½ cup)
½ cup sliced fresh mushrooms
1 bay leaf
1 cup low-sodium chicken broth

1 tablespoon flour
1 cup nonfat milk
1 to 2 sprigs fresh thyme, crushed without the stems
1/4 cup dried bread crumbs
1 tablespoon grated nonfat Parmesan cheese
Salt and freshly ground pepper

Heat a 5-quart saucepan over medium-high heat. Sauté the yellow and green onions, garlic, seafood, mushrooms, and bay leaf until the shrimp turns pink; stir frequently. Combine the broth, flour, milk, and thyme; mix well. Stir the milk mixture into the saucepan; stir constantly until the sauce thickens. Remove the saucepan from the heat. Remove the bay leaf.

Spray the bottom of a casserole with the cooking spray so that the ingredients will not stick to the bottom. Place the cooked pasta in the casserole. Pour the seafood sauce over the pasta. Sprinkle the bread crumbs and then the Parmesan cheese over the casserole. Salt and pepper the dish according to individual taste. Bake the casserole uncovered in a preheated oven at 350° for 15 minutes. Serve the hot dish immediately.

4 servings

Each serving provides:

248	Calories	34 g	Carbohydrate
24 g	Protein	252 mg	Sodium
2 g	Fat	79 mg	Cholesterol

100

Turkey Parmesan Casserole

Preparation time: 20 minutes
Baking time: 15 minutes
Preheat oven to 350°

A little turkey goes a long way! Subtly blended with the
flavor of Parmesan cheese, these tenderloin pieces of
turkey will make perfect sense over a heap of soft, warm
pasta. Pasta cooking is easy, elegant, and very flavorful
when combined with turkey, zucchini, and herbs. An
extra dash of paprika or cayenne will add a pleasant twist.

No stick cooking spray
2 cups (about 4 ounces) dry ribbon noodles, cooked
    according to package directions, drained, and rinsed
³/₄ pound extra-lean turkey, skinned, boned, and cut into
    tenderloin pieces (about 1 ¹/₂ cups)
1 small yellow onion, sliced into rings
¹/₂ cup julienned green onions
1 to 2 cloves garlic, crushed in a garlic press
1 cup sliced mushrooms
¹/₂ small zucchini, halved and sliced
1 tablespoon flour
1 cup nonfat milk
2 tablespoons grated nonfat Parmesan cheese
1 to 2 teaspoons minced fresh marjoram leaves

Salt and freshly ground pepper
Dash of paprika or cayenne pepper (optional,
   for a spicier dish)

Spray the bottom of a large, nonstick skillet and casserole
with the cooking spray so that the ingredients will not
stick to the bottom. Heat the skillet over medium-high
heat. In the skillet, evenly brown the turkey pieces to lock
in the juices; cook until golden brown, about 2 to 4 minutes per side. Add the yellow and green onions, garlic,
mushrooms, and zucchini. Sauté until the zucchini slices
are crisp-tender; stir frequently. Combine the flour, milk,
Parmesan cheese, and marjoram in a small bowl; mix well.
Stir the milk mixture into the skillet; stir constantly until
the sauce thickens.
   Place the cooked pasta in the casserole. Pour the
turkey sauce over the pasta. Salt and pepper the dish
according to individual taste. Bake the turkey in a preheated oven at 350° for 15 minutes. Garnish the dish with
paprika or cayenne. Serve the hot dish immediately.

4 servings

Each serving provides:

274	Calories	31 g	Carbohydrate
32 g	Protein	141 mg	Sodium
3 g	Fat	73 mg	Cholesterol

101

—✦—

Turkey and Mostaccioli Casserole

Preparation time: 20 minutes
Baking time: 15 minutes
Preheat oven to 350°

Turkey lovers looking for a simple, appetizing casserole
will enjoy using this recipe. Savor the subtle flavors of
turkey, mushrooms, and Parmesan along with a hint of
aromatic herbs. Of course, this superwonderful treat is
quick and easy to prepare.

No stick cooking spray
2 cups (about 4 ounces) dry mostaccioli pasta, cooked
    according to package directions, drained, and rinsed
³/₄ pound extra-lean ground turkey (about 1 ½ cups)
1 small yellow onion, sliced into rings
½ cup julienned green onions
1 to 2 cloves garlic, crushed in a garlic press
¼ to 1 small fresh anaheim chile, seeded, washed, and
    finely chopped (optional, for a spicier dish)
1 celery stalk with leaves, finely sliced
1 cup finely sliced fresh mushrooms
³/₄ cup low-sodium chicken or turkey broth
⅓ cup nonfat sour cream
1 to 2 teaspoons minced fresh marjoram leaves
3 tablespoons grated nonfat Monterey Jack cheese
Salt and freshly ground pepper

Spray the bottom of a large, nonstick skillet and casserole with the cooking spray so that the ingredients will not stick to the bottom.

Heat the skillet over medium-high heat. In the skillet, evenly brown the turkey for 5 minutes; stir frequently. Add the yellow and green onions, garlic, anaheim chile, celery, and mushrooms. Sauté until the celery is tender; stir frequently. Reduce the heat to low. Stir in the broth, sour cream, and marjoram. Simmer 2 minutes; stir occasionally.

Place the cooked pasta in the casserole. Pour the turkey sauce over the pasta; cover the pasta with the sauce. Sprinkle the cheese over the casserole. Salt and pepper the dish according to individual taste. Bake the casserole in a preheated oven at 350° for 15 minutes. Serve the hot dish immediately.

4 servings

Each serving provides:

297	Calories	30 g	Carbohydrate
35 g	Protein	188 mg	Sodium
4 g	Fat	63 mg	Cholesterol

Index

V